W9-AZA-665

Mind Over Body

Mind Over Body

The Key to Lasting Weight Loss
Is All in Your Head

Nordine Zouareg

Professional Fitness Coach at Miraval Spa & Resort

BROWNSBURG PUBLIC LIBRARY
450 SOUTH JEFFERSON STREET
BROWNSBURG, IN 46112

SPRINGBOARD PRESS

NEW YORK   BOSTON

To the strongest and most courageous people I know,

my mother and my father, Yamina and Naoui Zouareg

Copyright © 2007 by Nordine Zouareg

All rights reserved. Except as permitted under the U.S. Copyright Act of 1976, no part of this publication may be reproduced, distributed, or transmitted in any form or by any means, or stored in a database or retrieval system, without the prior written permission of the publisher.

Springboard Press
Hachette Book Group USA
237 Park Avenue, New York, NY 10017
Visit our Web site at www.HachetteBookGroupUSA.com

First Edition: June 2007

Springboard Press is an imprint of Grand Central Publishing. The Springboard name and logo are trademarks of Hachette Book Group USA.

Library of Congress Cataloging-in-Publication Data

Zouareg, Nordine.
    Mind over body : the key to lasting weight loss is all in your head / Nordine Zouareg.—1st ed.
        p. cm.
    ISBN 978-0-446-58077-9
    1. Weight loss—Psychological aspects. 2. Reducing exercises. 3. Mind and body. I. Title.
    RM222.2.Z794 2007
    613.2'5—dc22   2006019956

10 9 8 7 6 5 4 3 2 1

Photographs by Jerry Avenaim Photography Inc.
Book design and text composition by L&GMcRee

PRINTED IN THE UNITED STATES OF AMERICA

Contents

Acknowledgments

I thank from the bottom of my heart and the depth of my soul all the people who have contributed to this book and stood by me all the way. To Yogi Bhajan, for whose love and blessings I am forever grateful. To my wife, Keri, whose patience and love for me fueled my spirit when times were not so favorable. To my son, Armand, and my daughter, Isabella, for their daily dose of love, noise, and demands. To Dharma Singh Khalsa, MD, and Kirti Kaur Khalsa for their love, trust, and life-changing teachings. To my agent, Susan Ginsburg, and my editors, Karen Murgolo and Michelle Howry, for believing in me. To Judy Kern for helping me in the preparation of this book and for her wonderful spirit. To Jill Cohen, for trusting in the value of this book. To John and Maria Assaraf for inspiring me and supporting me with this project. To chef Cary Neff, who always believed in me and my work. To the amazing photographer Jerry Avenaim, whose creativity exceeded my expectations. To Liz Dickinson, CEO of Physi-Cal Enterprises, for her generosity and love.

Thanks also to Polly Anthony of Interscope Entertainment; Michelle Anthony; and Carol Berg, PsyD, for their constant love and appreciation. To Dana Paterson for seeing this book in her vision and for her warm encouragement. To my friends Dr. Ty Endean, Gurumeet Khalsa, Nirvair Khalsa, Jennifer Morris, Keith Arnold, Fred Singer, Beth Singer, Jeff Lamp, Alyson Steel, Mark Urlage, Matthew Hummel, Paul and Kathy Rizzuto, Bill Gower, Bret and April Bott, and Roger and Helen Abramson for their love and support. To Luz Elena Shearer, MS, RD, for her valuable feedback.

To all my friends and colleagues and the wonderful guests at Miraval Life in Balance—I am so grateful to have you in my life. Special thanks to Steve Case, Bill O'Donnell, George Ruff, and Joseph DeNucci, Miraval partners; and to Dan

Dearen, CFO, Dan Hirsch, vice president of business development, Harley Mayer-sohn, vice president of branding and marketing, and Chris Willett, executive assistant and director of projects, at Miraval, for their support and trust in me. My thanks also to Barbara MacDonald, public relations manager at Miraval, for making the photo shoot for this book run so smoothly.

Finally, to the thousands of clients and guests I've worked with throughout my career, you contributed to the creation of the concept for this book and don't even know it. Thank you for the great fun and for the life lessons I've gained from you.

Foreword

The Key to *Mind Over Body's* Success

I'll never forget the day I met Nordine, because it changed my life. I was working out on the upstairs balcony of Gold's Gym in Albuquerque, New Mexico. My trainer, a pretty buff dude himself, pointed to a strikingly handsome and obviously fit fellow downstairs and asked me, "How'd you like to meet Mr. Universe from Paris, France?"

I said I would very much like to meet him, so off we went downstairs. As Nordine and I shook hands that first time, we both felt the energy pass between us. It was as if we were each meeting a long-lost brother. That was the beginning of a wonderful friendship that continues to grow stronger with each passing day.

Not too long after, Nordine moved to Tucson, Arizona, and we began working together with patients in my Brain Longevity Program. We also started training together. Nordine, I learned, was a master at helping people lose fat, gain muscle, and regain their health fast and forever. I've seen him work wonders with people who came to our program out of shape and in dire need of physical fitness. In one particular instance that comes to mind, Suzy, a forty-eight-year-old patient, came to me with severe stress-related memory loss. Nordine quickly isolated her physical problem and designed a specific fitness program that helped heal her mind as it strengthened her body.

The Benefits of a *Mind Over Body* Lifestyle

When you follow the exercise and nutritional ideas in this book, you will definitely feel great. Your mind will be sharp and refreshed, your muscles will feel invigorated, and your joints will be fluid.

But, of course, "feeling better" is a subjective assessment. As a doctor who respects science, I'd like to share with you some of the many well-researched scientific benefits of the mind/body exercise plan presented in *Mind Over Body*.

Let's begin with your skin. Many people today, men and women alike, spend millions of dollars on potions and lotions to make their skin look beautiful. But true beauty, as I'm sure you'll agree, must come from the inside, and Nordine's program gives you a distinctive, healthy glow. I think you'll notice it right away.

Next, recent research clearly shows that exercise can actually keep the brain, as well as the body, young. When you follow a plan like *Mind Over Body*, which includes techniques such as visualization and meditation, depression is eased, anxiety is reduced, and memory improves. Work by my colleague Andrew Newberg, MD, at the Center for Spirituality and the Mind at the University of Pennsylvania School of Medicine, where I am a research fellow, has shown that both these practices help your brain to function at a much higher level.

Moreover, fascinating new work by Dr. Sara Lazar at Harvard has revealed an actual antiaging effect of meditation. The thickness of the cortical, or outside, layer of the brain increases with ongoing practice. This remarkable discovery shows how the brain can be changed positively throughout life.

Studies also indicate that people who are at risk for Alzheimer's disease because of genetics or family history score better on memory tests when they exercise. Moreover, my own research shows an improvement in attention, concentration, and focus, as well as an anti-Alzheimer's effect, when you follow the mind/body principles, such as daily meditation, that Nordine shares in this book.

Equally significant, following the *Mind Over Body* plan will normalize your sleep pattern and help you sleep more deeply. This is particularly meaningful because, according to the latest research, close to 60 percent of Americans report that they don't sleep well.

As you're probably aware, heart disease is still America's number one killer of both men and women, which is why it's important to note that the exercise and nutritional plans in this book will also reduce your risk for heart disease and stroke by building a healthy cardiovascular system, normalizing your blood pressure, and balancing your good and bad cholesterol levels. At the same time, your lung function will be markedly improved, and if you're a smoker, your habit will go up in smoke!

And what about your bones? Nordine's exercise plan will increase bone density, which will reduce your risk for osteoporosis and the bone loss associated with menopause. You will also have increased joint mobility, improved flexibility, and better balance, all of which are especially important as you reach midlife. Many of us plan on living well into our eighties and beyond, so building strong bones is important to reduce the chances of falls and disability.

Exercise also enhances your immune function, and there is even some preliminary evidence to support the idea that an exercise program like Nordine's may help to reduce the risk of breast, colon, prostate, and other cancers. A recent study, in fact, reveals a number of improvements in survivors of breast cancer who exercise regularly.

When you put the *Mind Over Body* program to work in your life, your digestion and elimination will improve. I remember once hearing that if you exercise well, you can even digest stones! I wouldn't recommend trying it, but you get the message: Exercise is good for your gastrointestinal system.

And because you will simply feel better and younger in all areas of your body, your libido will also be boosted. As your overall health and vitality improve, you will look and feel more attractive, and you'll have greater self-esteem, less stress, and more energy than you could have imagined.

There are three more important benefits to note. One is that Nordine's mind/body/spirit approach will cause your spiritual well-being to soar. Spirituality is an important component of a happy life and leads to one of higher quality and meaning.

Second, when you take care of yourself in this way, you will increase your net worth. How can that be? you might ask. When you're functioning at a higher level physically, mentally, and spiritually, all the good things in the universe are drawn to you, including wealth. And don't forget that when you're healthy, happy, and whole as a human being, you simply don't spend so much money on health care. That puts more money in your pocket, be it for getting out of debt, saving for retirement, putting the kids through school, or whatever your financial needs might be.

But perhaps the best benefit of all is this plan's proven success in the long term. The program in *Mind Over Body* is the only one I know of whose benefits have been clinically proved to be long-lasting. Unlike other programs that merely show you how to lose the weight, Nordine's gives you a proven way to *keep it off.* I believe the main reason the *Mind Over Body* program is so effective in the long term is that it taps into your core desire. The ideas presented in this book become so embedded in your true identity that they become second nature to you. The concepts become your lifestyle as you effortlessly manifest the optimal health and fitness that are your destiny.

The Secret of *Mind Over Body*

At the heart of *Mind Over Body* is one powerful, unique message: Nordine will teach you how to use your *mind* to tap into your inner power of peak performance. In addition to well-known techniques such as visualization, which Nordine used to become a world champion, he also recommends mind/body techniques such as meditation and mental reconditioning, which are generally associated with Eastern spiritual traditions but have not, until now, been applied to teaching true lifelong health and fitness. The techniques he presents and teaches in this book are those he learned from Yogi Bhajan, the highest yoga master of our generation.

These mind/body exercises are also steeped in medical science. They have been shown to have a positive effect on every system of the body and to help heal every illness ever studied, from diabetes to chronic pain. Equally important, however, they're unbeatable for helping you focus your mind, relax your body, and get in touch with your inner being.

I'll never forget the day Nordine and I went to visit the master himself. The yogi looked at Nordine with his deep, luminous, penetrating eyes, which seemed to see the past, present, and future all at once.

"You're an avatar," the yogi said to Mr. Universe. An avatar is someone who is ahead of his time, and the yogi recognized that in Nordine.

"Sir, I want to write a book," Nordine said.

"Just relax," the master said. "Write from the heart."

I believe with all my heart that Nordine listened very well. He has written a book from his heart, and I know it will take you on a wonderful journey to a lifetime of fitness and great health.

You deserve it. Enjoy the blessing.

Dharma Singh Khalsa, MD
President/Medical Director
Alzheimer's Prevention Foundation
www.drdharma.com
Tucson, Arizona

Mind Over Body

Introduction

The Path to Fitness—Mine and Yours

*Your body is the servant of your mind and has no choice
but to obey your thoughts.*

I don't believe that anyone who claims to be a leader can ask people to follow him—whether the journey takes them from New York to Chicago or from self-doubt and poor health to confidence and fitness—unless he's traveled that path himself. I've traveled every inch of the journey you'll be making with me in this book. And my path, like many of yours, has been strewn with stumbling blocks and disrupted by detours. In fact, it's because I was able to surmount those obstacles to arrive at the place where I am now that I know I can lead you, too, to a place where your body, mind, and spirit will work together to give you a healthier, happier life.

The beginning of my life was not auspicious. In fact, my mother used to tell me that I "died" three times as an infant. It was only because of her perseverance (and some inborn luck or stubbornness within me) that I survived to celebrate my first birthday. I was born on July 1, 1962, to illiterate Bedouin parents in the back of a French army truck in Algeria. My mother was just fifteen years old, and my father was twenty-nine. Algeria was a French colony at the time, and the truck was part of a convoy taking Bedouins to vote on the question of Algerian independence.

As they were traveling through the desert, my mother went into labor, and the driver finally had to stop the truck so that she could deliver her baby by the side of the road with the help of the elder women of the tribe. I weighed just over two pounds at birth, and my mother later told me that all she could see of me were my eyes and my stomach. I was literally nothing but skin and bones, and to this day it amazes me that I survived that journey, much less all that was to come after. My mother—young and ignorant but determined—managed to keep me alive.

We lived in a small town called El Houamed, which was the last oasis before entering the Sahara. To my mother, living a difficult life in the desert, I presented a terrible dilemma. No more than a child herself, she was burdened with a sickly baby who no one—including she—believed would survive. Finally, after about six months, the elder women held a "wisdom meeting," which would, to put it bluntly, decide my fate. The problem, as they saw it, was essentially this: We don't think this baby will survive, but we can't kill him, so what are we going to do? In their "wisdom," they decided that my mother should make sure I was fed and happy, then leave me on a tombstone in the cemetery and walk away. But if she heard me cry, the elder women cautioned, she would have to take me back.

My mother did what the women said. She fed me and left me on a tombstone. She has said that I seemed content. But the minute she turned her back to walk away, I began to cry. Of course, she went back for me.

A few weeks later, my parents decided to take me to M'Sila, a larger town about three hours north of where we lived, to get me proper medical care. They took me to the main hospital in the center of M'Sila and left me with the doctors overnight for observation. When my mother went back to the hospital the next day, the doctor who had been treating me told her I was dead. My mother asked to see my body, but the doctor refused.

In fact, I was not dead, but my vital signs were at such a dangerous level that the doctor and his colleagues honestly believed they wouldn't be able to save me. To them, I was as good as dead. On the one hand, they believed that keeping me alive would only cause my mother more pain when I ultimately died—as they were sure I would. On the other hand, they understood that if she knew I was still alive, she would continue trying to save me. And so, when my mother asked to see my body, the doctor believed he had no choice but to refuse.

My mother, however, wouldn't leave M'Sila without seeing me, so she went to the police for assistance. An officer returned with her to the hospital and told the doctor that she had every right to claim her baby's body and give him a proper burial. At that point, there was nothing for the doctor to do but to confess that I was not dead—yet. He apologized profusely but said that he truly believed he had done the right thing. As he saw it, my mother was very young—she could have more children—and letting me die in what he considered a "proper" place would be easier for her than watching me die in the desert.

So once more my mother took me back home, but both my parents knew I was in critical need of immediate medical attention. Their last resort, they felt, was to take me to France. All Algerians were at that time still French citizens. But my parents spoke only Berber, and they didn't have any money for the trip. Still, they managed to collect what they needed from their fellow tribespeople and, speaking not a word of French, set out to build a new life for themselves and me in France.

There I was promptly diagnosed with rickets. The French doctors treated me in the hospital and then sent me home. But my health problems continued for the next several years.

My father worked whatever jobs he could find to support our family, which grew to a total of thirteen children—me, three brothers, and nine sisters—all living in a small two-bedroom apartment. In addition to economic difficulties, we also had to deal with extreme prejudice against all North Africans. In school I was beaten up regularly and had my lunch and clothing stolen. Thinking back on it now, I realize that I was a skinny runt of a kid with absolutely no self-esteem. In some terrible way, the negative energy I was putting out was almost certainly exacerbating the treatment I received. That insight, however, was a long time in coming; at the time all I knew was that I was miserable.

The turning point came when I arrived home from high school one day to find my entire family gathered around the television. They were watching a gymnastics competition, including one guy performing the iron cross on the still rings—a pair of rings suspended from the ceiling about eight feet above the floor. The iron cross requires the gymnast to hold on to the rings with his arms straight out at his sides while both his body and the rings remain absolutely still. The amount of upper body strength required to hold this position is enormous. The guy who was doing it wasn't big, but he was "ripped" and symmetrical. At that moment, I knew I wanted to be that gymnast.

Although I didn't realize it then, I'd stumbled upon the single most powerful tool for any athlete—or anyone trying to get healthy and lose weight: visualization.

Normally, if you visualize yourself in a particular situation, it takes a while for that visualization to become internalized and move from your conscious to your subconscious mind. But that afternoon, I claimed that image on the TV screen for myself. The picture of me as strong and powerful immediately became anchored in my subconscious, and I knew I would one day make it a reality.

An *anchor* is a specific stimulus that calls forth particular thoughts and emotions. When you anchor something, it's like falling in love. It doesn't happen on a conscious, rational level; rather, your heart speaks to your mind, and you know it is right. Once the anchor is in place, it will always be there for you to call upon to reinforce your commitment if and when you feel yourself wavering. In that moment, I fell in love with the concept of being and feeling like that young man on the still rings. Doing that became my core desire, and having that desire unleashed a magic within me that I couldn't possibly have known I had.

You must understand that I was then nineteen years old. I weighed 108 pounds. My younger sisters were bigger than I was. But once I had identified my core desire, I became unstoppable. I saw myself having the body of that gymnast on TV, and that image allowed me to use the power of my intention, which was to learn whatever I needed to learn in order to fulfill my desire. At that point, I took what I believed to be an appropriate action: I went to a gym to learn gymnastics.

I joined a local gym that had a gymnastics team, of which three of my friends were already members. Because my friends were good gymnasts, I was allowed to join the team as a favor to them. For a while, I was just too skinny. While my teammates were performing more and more difficult moves, I was doing bench presses in a corner with an empty bar because that was all I could lift.

Eventually, however, the coach took me aside and told me that if I ever hoped to succeed at gymnastics or any other sport, I needed to put on some weight. And so I went in search of a weight lifting gym. I remember walking in and seeing the owner/instructor coming toward me. He looked like a mountain that was growing bigger with each step he took in my direction. I turned and walked out. But my true core desire was still there.

My parents had always been very supportive of whatever I wanted to do, but they had also always made it clear that getting an education was going to be my key to a better life. I never gave up on education—in fact, I later earned a master's degree in physical education—but I also knew that if I didn't achieve my core desire, my education wasn't going to help me. I applied my resolve and returned to the gym.

I worked out six days a week for about an hour each day, and I asked a lot of questions. Whenever I saw someone in the gym who was more bulked up and muscular than I was, I asked him what he had done to get that way. I learned the proper ways to eat and work out, and slowly my core desire began to shift. I no longer wanted to be that gymnast; I wanted to be a competitive bodybuilder, and the image I now held in my mind was that of the bodybuilder I saw myself becoming. I began building my body and, at the same time, became more resolved than ever to succeed. The more successful I became, the better I felt about myself. My successes were continually fueling my desire.

Three years later, in 1986, I won four bodybuilding titles—Mr. France, Mr. Europe, Mr. World, and Mr. Universe. But my initial success actually derailed me. My original goal had been to get out of my misery and find happiness through bodybuilding, but I now became miserably obsessed with my body.

I was constantly driven by the fear that I wouldn't be good enough, that I wouldn't win, that my fans would desert me. Truthfully, if you spend all day staring at your body and measuring your body fat, you don't have much time left over to devote to your mental and emotional well-being. And if you're afraid all the time, there's no way you can be happy. Since that time, I've come to understand that unhappiness is something we create for ourselves when we stop trusting what comes from within and lose touch with our true core desire. For a while, I lost track of that, and I needed to rediscover my inner truth.

In 1995 I came to the United States and settled in Albuquerque, New Mexico. There I met Dr. Dharma Singh Khalsa, a medical doctor, yogi, and author. Dr. Khalsa is the president and medical director of the Alzheimer's Prevention Foundation, and I credit him with turning my life around for the second time.

I began to work with Dr. Khalsa as his personal trainer; it was a wonderful experience for both of us. As I coached him to make his body stronger, he taught me yoga and meditation, through which I was finally able to get out of my body-obsessed mind-set.

In 1998 Dr. Khalsa invited me to join his company, Khalsa International, and become fitness director at the facility in Tucson, Arizona, where he treats his patients. He also introduced me to Joseph DeNucci, then the general manager at Miraval resort, whose "life in balance" philosophy was—and is—so in tune with my own. While I was working at Khalsa International, Mr. DeNucci, who had been a yoga teacher and is a very spiritual person, invited me to come to Miraval for a couple of days to see if I would like to create a fitness program for the spa. After those two days, my energy was flowing, and I knew in my heart that it was a place I'd be staying for a very long time.

My journey has taught me many things: that harnessing the power of a true core desire can change your entire life; that being physically fit and healthy must go hand in hand with being mentally and emotionally healthy; that if you want other people to love you, you first have to love yourself; and finally that loving what you're doing creates a positive flow of energy that's contagious. If you're passionate about your life, other people will share that passion.

A New Approach to Fitness

In the pages that follow, I will lead you on your own journey so that you, too, can arrive at a place where your mind and emotions are driving your desire to lose weight and become fit on both a conscious and a subconscious level. You will be using your mind to direct your body and working toward fitness from the inside out. As a result, I can promise that you *will* become thin, trim, fit, and as beautiful on the outside as you are on the inside.

There are many books on many subjects, including physical fitness, that tell people *what* to do. In my opinion, that is a lot like writing on someone else's blackboard with your own chalk. What I mean is that the authors of these books want you to see things from their perspective. In contrast, I will be asking you to consider your own perspective and to decide whether shifting the way you see yourself in relation to the world might serve you better. I believe that most of us already know what we should be doing to lose weight and improve fitness. In fact, with all the information on exercise and nutrition coming at us from the media every day, it would be almost impossible *not* to know. The problem is that for most people, there's a large disconnect between knowledge and action. My goal is to teach you how to shift your thoughts so that you are able to go from *knowing* to *doing*.

In this book, I will take you through the very same steps I followed to arrive at where I am today mentally, emotionally, and physically. I will provide all the information you need about what kinds of foods to eat and what kinds of exercise programs will work for you to achieve your individual goal and level of fitness. But that's part two of the plan. First I'm going to provide you with the information and understanding you need to be able to follow through with my program and actually achieve what you want.

The bottom line is that goals are achieved when the right information is loaded into the subconscious part of your brain. I will teach you how to harness the power of your subconscious mind to build the fit and fabulous body you want but have never been able to achieve. It's a question of *mind over body!*

Before we begin, I want to point out that my professional expertise lies in helping people to achieve health and fitness, which is, of course, the focus of this book. Personally, however, I know that all the information I'll be giving you can be used to achieve whatever you truly desire in every aspect of your life. All of these techniques are designed to create the right balance of body, mind, and spirit, which is all anyone needs to banish stress, defeat fear, overcome failure, and bring more happiness into his or her life.

THE FOUR STEPS
FROM KNOWING
TO DOING

One

Identify Your Core Desire

People spend most of their time thinking about what they don't want and then wondering why it keeps showing up over and over again in their lives.

Beth was an attractive brunette who appeared to be in her early forties. She came into my office at Miraval for a consultation, sat down, and immediately told me that she wanted to lose thirty pounds. When I asked her why, she replied that she wanted to fit into her clothes and to look better than her ex-husband's girlfriend. As we continued to talk, it soon became clear that every time she looked in the mirror, she felt fat, unattractive, and insecure, and she simply didn't want to feel that way anymore.

I asked if she had children. *Yes, two—ten and eight.* Are they healthy? *Oh, well, you know, they're like every other kid.* But not all kids are sick. Are they healthy? *Well, we have a babysitter, and she calls in for food, so . . .* Well, I knew what that meant. They were eating pizza and burgers and parking themselves in front of the television every day after school.

As Beth was talking, I noticed that she kept repeating one phrase: "I'm overweight." I started writing down how many times she said it.

At the end of our session, Beth looked at me and asked, "So what do I do now?" At that point, I handed her the piece of paper I'd been filling with notes. When she saw how many times she'd said, "I'm overweight," she was astonished. "Did I really say that so many times?" she asked.

I told Beth that she'd been using her mind to affirm to her body that she was fat. Because your body is the servant of your mind, it has no choice but to listen. If your body listens to your mind telling it how overweight you are, your body is not going to work to make you thin and fit; it's going to work to do exactly the opposite—keep you overweight. It's simply what your mind has been telling it to do.

Then I suggested that we take another look at the reasons she'd given for wanting to lose weight: to fit into her clothes and to look better than her ex-husband's girlfriend. How did she think she would feel when she'd achieved those goals? Listening to her tone of voice and watching her expression as she told me how she'd feel, I could tell that, although she certainly had strong feelings attached to those goals, they weren't deep enough, passionate enough, or—most important—positive enough to create the kinds of changes she truly needed and wanted to make.

What Beth really needed was to search more deeply within herself for a real reason to reach her weight-loss goal. She needed a reason that would generate the kinds of powerful, positive feelings that would tell me—and most of all her—that this was more than just a reason, that it was, in fact, her core desire. Perhaps, I suggested, her core desire was to turn her life around; to be truly happy instead of insecure; to be a role model for her children.

Finally, I had hit a chord. When she thought about how she'd feel once she had achieved those goals, she was literally in tears. For her, this was a truly inspirational aha moment. She was able to see that instead of using negative reasons to lose weight, which were creating negative energy, she could act from a positive reason fueled by a true core desire to be happy and to make a better life for herself and her children, and that this would release the positive mental and emotional energy (the magic) she had within her to achieve her physical goal.

After that, I worked with Beth not only to create a nutrition and exercise program that she could realistically follow but also to help her take the key steps necessary to guarantee that her program would become as habitual as getting up in the morning and brushing her teeth. I made it clear that this would take some effort on her part and that after she left Miraval, she'd have to keep at it for four to six weeks until her routine became automatic. But I assured her that after thirty to forty days, it would be something she'd continue to do without even having to think about it.

In the weeks after she went back home, Beth phoned me a couple of times to report that she was sticking to her resolve. After four months, she called to let me know that she'd lost twenty-five pounds and was homing in on her goal weight. Not only that, but she was feeling so positive about herself that she was also determined to change the way her children were eating and spending their time after school.

Do You Really Want to Change?

No one can "make" another person change his or her behavior. Only you can control your choices and create that change. All I can do for you in this book is what I do when I'm sitting in a room with a client—to help you determine what your goals are and what you truly want for yourself, identify your current negative and positive behaviors, and create a plan of action that will facilitate the changes you want to make. Doing all that is a process—one that I go through with my clients every day and that I will be going through with you as well. The first step, which we'll learn about in this chapter, is to identify your core desire—the self-generated, internal need that will motivate you finally to change.

Change doesn't happen in an instant. In fact, most of us, at least initially, are afraid of change. If you don't believe me, just think how many people remain for years in dead-end jobs or moribund marriages. Why? Because they may not be happy with the result of their current behavior, but at least they know what that result is. And they're afraid that if they change their behavior, the result may be worse. Even our bodies hate to change. All our systems and our organs work constantly to keep things the same. What our bodies seek is *homeostasis*—the maintenance of internal stability. That's a biological fact.

So how do we bring about change for ourselves, mentally and physically? Change is, as I've said, a process. We move from not thinking about change at all to thinking about it, planning it, and then testing various means of creating it.

Since you're reading this book, you may at least have reached the point of thinking about change. To move past that point, you need to ask yourself three questions:

- Why do I want to change my behavior (the pros)? (For example: I want to feel better about myself. I want to look better. I want to do everything I can to live better longer. I want to set a good example for my kids. I want my husband to stop nagging me.)

- Why shouldn't I try to change my behavior (the cons)? (For example: I'm so busy already that I don't need any more stress in my life. I don't want to be a failure. It's going to be hard for me to be with my friends and stick to my healthy eating plan. The rest of my family isn't going to want to eat this way, so I'll be cooking two meals.)
- Do my pros outweigh my cons? (Only you can answer that question!)

If your answer to the last question is yes, you're at the point of being interested in change. Being interested, however, isn't a strong enough feeling or motivation to get you where you think you want to be. If you're merely interested, you're not committed, and you'll most likely give up as soon as you encounter an obstacle or challenge.

Being interested means you'll do what's convenient; being committed means you'll do whatever it takes. Let's say you're thinking about something as simple as changing your hairstyle. You're interested, but you're not committed. Chances are the minute someone questions the idea, or if you can't get an appointment right away, you'll drop the whole thing and move on to some other "interest."

The Power of the Subconscious

In a moment, I'll begin taking you through the steps that will lead you to discover and connect with your own true core desire. But first it's important for you to understand the power of the subconscious mind so that you will see how Beth's constantly telling herself she was fat was actually causing her to be fat, and how your own subconscious beliefs about yourself may be preventing you from achieving your own most deeply held desires.

Your subconscious mind accounts for 83 percent of your brain mass and is responsible for 98 percent of your perceptions and behaviors, including habits and beliefs, memory, personality, and self-image. It cannot tell the truth from a lie or the real from the imagined. It accepts as true every thought or image you send it.

The ideas that are fixed in your subconscious have been determined by your education, conditioning, and repetition. They involve all your senses, and they affect every aspect of your present behavior. If, for example, every time you look in the mirror you're focusing on how fat you are, you will subconsciously be affirming your fatness to yourself, and the consequence of that subconscious affirmation is that your daily behaviors will be directed toward fulfilling what you believe about yourself. In the following chapters, I'll teach you how to replace those negative subconscious affirmations with positive ones that will lead you to achieve what you *do* want instead of keeping you stuck in what you *don't* want.

To show how your subconscious may be driving your behavior and perceptions, imagine that you have a subconscious memory attached to a particular scent or aroma. It could be anything from the scent of your mother's favorite perfume to the smell of burning wood. If your mother's perfume reminds you of her coming to kiss you good night, it has a positive connotation. If it reminds you of her going out in the evening and leaving you home alone, it has a negative connotation. The same goes for the smell of burning wood. If it reminds you of happy family evenings in front of the fireplace, that's good. If you were once trapped in a burning building, that's bad. Now imagine that you're in the middle of a conversation with someone, and suddenly you smell that same perfume or burning wood. If your subconscious memory is favorable, the conversation you are having will strike you as positive. But if your associations are negative, the conversation will take a wrong turn. You won't know why—you certainly won't associate the outcome with what you smelled—but your subconscious mind will be affecting what's happening in your life at the moment.

By the same token, if something in your past has led you to believe (on a subconscious level) that you are fat or are a couch potato, you will, without realizing it, be making your outward behavior conform to your inner beliefs. Let's say, for example, that your mother used sweet treats to bribe you to behave well. Your subconscious has been programmed to associate sweets with a reward. You may be able to override those beliefs temporarily by using your willpower, but over time your internal beliefs will always be stronger than your willpower. To create any permanent change in behavior, you must first change your negative inner beliefs. Failing to do that is why so many people who go on a diet or start an exercise program ultimately gain back all the weight they lose or simply stop exercising.

The good news is that you can bring your subconscious thoughts and beliefs into consciousness, and once you are able to do that, you can change them. Keep reading and I'll help you to do just that.

Listen to Yourself

What I'll be asking you to do first is an essential part of the process of getting to know yourself, understanding the underlying beliefs that have been driving your behavior, and finding the deep-seated desire that will create your commitment to change. Before you start, however, I'm going to ask you to commit to taking the time to look deep within yourself and answer the following questions as fully, openly, and honestly as you can.

The problem for many people is that they've become so used to looking outward for validation and satisfaction that they've lost touch with their ability to look inward. So if you've been telling yourself that you "need" or "ought" to lose weight—because, for example, society tells you it's better to be thin, because a fitness trainer tells you to do it, or even because a doctor tells you'll be healthier if you exercise more—I'm here to tell you that you've been looking for motivation in all the wrong places. Your behavior has always been your choice; it is generated from within. No one else has made you behave the way you do, and changing your behavior must also be your choice, because no one else can make you change or impose a reason to change on you.

You may have been listening to other people for a very long time: your parents, your spouse, your friends and coworkers, or the many "experts" you see or hear or whose opinions you read or hear in the media every day. You may even have determined what you "think" other people want you to do without their ever having voiced an opinion.

It may be that when you were a kid, you thought you knew it all and didn't listen to anyone. But then, as time went on, you became much more attached to the opinions of others. You may even have gotten to the point where you believe that the opinions of others are more important than your own. Now is the time to begin listening to yourself again, because whatever is going on in the world around you is not nearly as important to you and your future as what's going on inside you.

A true core desire is not something you get from without; it's something you already have. In other words, if you are waiting for me or anyone else to provide you with the motivation you lack for changing your behavior, you might as well stop reading right now. It is not within my power to motivate you. It is, however, within my power to help you discover motivation within yourself, and the strongest motivation there is, is your own true core desire. It's there, it's probably the most powerful untapped resource each one of us has, and once you learn to access it, the riches will flow freely and forever.

The really good news is that if you follow the steps I provide to identify your core desire and develop a plan for reaching it, you *can* and *will* reprogram your subconscious mind—and once you do that, your body *will* follow.

To begin getting back in touch with your own true feelings so that you will be able to reap the benefits of that inner wealth, let's begin with this simple but revealing exercise.

1. Write down the most serious crisis in your life right now, whether it's money, health, relationships, or a combination of things. Whatever you see as a crisis has the potential to affect your health and wellness.

_____

_____

_____

_____

2. Write down the one word that best describes how you feel when you think of this crisis. It could be anxious, depressed, miserable, fearful, helpless, hopeless, ugly, ashamed, discouraged, worthless, guilty, vulnerable, hurt, inadequate, afraid, weak—whatever comes up for you.

_____

3. Now write down the one word that best describes how you'd feel if that crisis no longer existed. You can use words such as happy, peaceful, hopeful, trustworthy, beautiful, strong, or relaxed—any word of your choosing.

_____

4. Take a minute or so to reflect on that word and the feeling attached to it. It is how you will feel when you have achieved your core desire. Acknowledge that it is your birthright to feel that way. It is how you can feel every day of your life if you chose to. Now describe that feeling.

_____

_____

_____

_____

_____

_____

_____

I want you to remember the feeling you just had when you completed step 4 of this exercise, because it's also the feeling that will let you know when you've identified your core desire.

The Three Steps to Discovering and Connecting with Your Core Desire

Now that you have some sense of what you're seeking, it's time to dig a bit deeper to discover the core desire that will motivate and inspire you to change once and for all. With that in mind, find a quiet place and a time when you won't be interrupted. The best time, I have found, is shortly after awaking, before your mind becomes occupied with all the day's activities. If that isn't possible for you, do it whenever you are likely to be left undisturbed. To help clear your mind of all the external chatter you've been listening to for so long, do the following deep-breathing exercise.

- Make yourself comfortable.
- Inhale deeply and hold the breath for 3 seconds. Exhale and repeat this process 3 times.
- Roll your neck gently forward and to the left side, then forward again and to the right side—not backward, which would put pressure on the back of your neck. Repeat this 10 times. Breathe through your nose, inhaling as you move your head to the right and exhaling as you move it to the left. Repeat this exercise 5 times on each side.

Now you're ready to begin.

Step One: Evaluate Your Current Health and Wellness

Seven-time Tour de France winner and cancer survivor Lance Armstrong asks, "What are you dying from that stops you from achieving your dreams?" To find out what might be impeding you, complete the three sentences in each of the following areas, then circle one of the four "satisfaction levels" in each area.

1.   Physical Health

My current physical health is: _____

(Are you satisfied with the state of your health? Is there anything about your health that you'd like to improve? Do you have a particular problem or problems you could improve with changes in lifestyle and diet?)

My current belief about my physical health is:

_____

_____

_____

_____

(Do you feel that you've taken control of your health? Have you given in to feeling less than well because you don't know how to make yourself feel better? Do you believe you're as healthy as you can possibly be?)

My current physical health pattern is:

_____

_____

_____

_____

(Do you sail through the cold and flu season without getting sick? Do you seem to catch whatever is going around? Do you try to take better care of yourself, to exercise and eat healthily, and then quit because it just seems too hard?)

I am doing great.   *I am satisfied.*   *I am okay.*   *I need help.*

2. Fitness Level

My current fitness or activity level is: _____

(Do you engage in any regular physical activity—from walking to tap dancing to bike riding? Do you take the stairs instead of the elevator whenever possible? Do you just move from your car to your desk and back again?)

My current belief about my fitness is:

_____

_____

_____

_____

(Do you think you're as fit as you can possibly be? Would you like to have more energy, strength, and stamina? Are you unhappy with your level of fitness but believe there's nothing you can do to improve it?)

My current exercise or activity pattern is:

_____

_____

_____

_____

(Do you get all revved up and decide you're going to exercise regularly and then stop after a while? Do you get more active when the weather's nice and you can be outdoors, then go into hibernation for the winter? Are you more or less active now than you were five years ago?)

I am doing great.   *I am satisfied.*   *I am okay.*   *I need help.*

3.   Height and Body Weight

My current height and body weight are: _____

My current belief about my body weight is:

_____

_____

_____

_____

(Do you think your weight is about right for your age, height, and bone structure? Do you think it's within your power to control it? Compared to your friends, how would you describe your body weight? Would you want to lose weight if you could? If you think you can't, what do you believe is keeping you from doing it?)

My current eating pattern is:

_____

_____

_____

_____

(Do you think you eat healthily most, all, or none of the time? Do you eat pretty well at home but splurge when you eat out? Do you eat well during the week and pig out on weekends?)

I am doing great.   *I am satisfied.*   *I am okay.*   *I need help.*

4. Stress Management

My current stress level is: _____

(How much stress is related to your current job—not much, some, a lot, more than you can handle? Do you get to relax once you're at home, or do you bring your work stress with you? Do you wake up already feeling stressed, or do you have trouble sleeping because you take your stress to bed with you?)

My current belief about my stress level is:

_____

_____

_____

_____

(Do you think your stress is just a part of life and there's not much you can do about it? Do you think you help to create some of your own stress? Do you see that if you were able to change a couple of things in your life, your stress would go down? If so, do you know how you could be making those changes, or do you believe they're beyond your control?)

My current level of stress management is:

_____

_____

_____

_____

(Do you think you have your stress under control? Do you feel overwhelmed much or all of the time? Do you have a way to relax and "dump" your stress when you feel that it's becoming too much?)

I am doing great.   *I am satisfied.*   *I am okay.*   *I need help.*

Here's how Nancy, a top executive at an accounting firm in Chicago and mother of two, answered these questions.

My current physical health is: *Poor*

My current belief about my physical health is:

My parents both had heart problems. I am genetically predisposed to have heart disease. It's in the family.

My current physical health pattern is:

I don't really pay attention to my health because I am too busy and have no time to do so. I have high blood pressure and am taking medication to control it. I also take medication to stabilize my thyroid.

I am doing great.   *I am satisfied.*   *I am okay.*   I need help.

My current fitness or activity level is: *Light*

My current belief about my fitness is:

No matter what I do, I cannot stand being at the gym with all those fit people. They all look like they came out of a fitness magazine. I prefer to walk outside.

My current exercise or activity pattern is:

I try to walk one mile on Saturdays and Sundays if I don't have other things to do.

I am doing great.   *I am satisfied.*   I am okay.   *I need help.*

My current height and body weight are: *5'2" and 150 pounds*

My current belief about my body weight is:

I am fat. I don't like my stomach or my legs, and my entire body seems fat. I can't seem to lose weight. I've tried everything, and it didn't really work. I lose a few pounds, then I stop and regain the weight. I feel hopeless. It is hard to be on a diet and hard to be at the gym every day.

My current eating pattern is:

I try to watch what I eat. I'm not hungry in the morning, so I eat two meals on most days—one big meal at lunch and another at dinner. I don't really read food labels because I eat out most of the time. When I grocery shop, I mostly buy food for the kids: lunch packs, snacks for school, etc.

> *I am doing great.*   *I am satisfied.*   *I am okay.*   *I need help.*

My current stress level is: *High*

My current belief about my stress level is:

I have no choice; I have to make a living and raise my kids. I feel like if I stopped doing what I do and the way I do it, I'd lose the momentum and would not be effective anymore. It feels as if this is a "high" for me. That is the way I am—a high-energy woman.

My current level of stress management is:

I feel overwhelmed at work and in my personal life. I work more than 12 hours a day. When I get home, I cook dinner for my husband and two kids. I clean and organize my home after work. I work on the computer for a few hours at night. I go to bed at around 11 p.m., and I wake up at 5 a.m., get the kids fed, and take them to school.

> *I am doing great.*   *I am satisfied.*   *I am okay.*   *I need help.*

BROWNSBURG PUBLIC LIBRARY

If you circled *I am doing great* or *I am satisfied* in any area, you probably *are* doing great. If you circled *I am okay* or *I need help,* you need to take a close look at your inner beliefs and see how they may be preventing you from doing better. If, for example, you are constantly telling yourself that you're fat, that belief is going to translate into behavior that will guarantee that you remain what you believe you are—overweight. If you believe that you don't have time to exercise, well, guess what?

Once you see how this works, it's time to move on and list your goals, particularly for those areas where you're less than satisfied with your current situation.

Step Two: Identify Your Physical Health, Fitness, Weight-Loss, and Stress Management Goals

Once you've completed step one, you've identified those areas in your life where you could be doing better—those marked "I am okay"—and those where you know you need help. Now's the time to determine what your goals are in terms of improving those areas.

In step two, you simply write down what you want to achieve in terms of fitness and weight loss in each of the four areas you've already evaluated. Think of as many goals as you can for each category and jot them down in random order. Here are some typical answers.

- I want to get my blood pressure down.
- I want to get my cholesterol under control.
- I want to be able to climb the stairs without getting out of breath.
- I want to play hoops with my kid without getting winded.
- I want to lose twenty pounds.
- I want to fit into my size 6 jeans.
- I want to weigh what I did when I graduated from college.
- I want to get rid of my bulging tummy (or gut).
- I want to be firm again instead of flabby.
- I want to feel exhilarated, not exhausted, at the end of the day.
- I want to get organized and not feel so stressed all the time.

Now that you see how it works, it's your turn.

1. Physical health goals:

_____

_____

_____

_____

2. Fitness goals:

_____

_____

_____

_____

3. Weight-loss goals:

_____

_____

_____

_____

4. Stress management goals:

_____

_____

_____

_____

So now you know what your goals are. Goals, however, are just that—an expression of purpose. Goals are important because they're clear, specific, pragmatic, and measurable in their attainment. But to achieve a goal, whatever it may be, you need something more. You need to discover the deeper purpose behind that goal, which is your *core desire.*

Without identifying and connecting with a positive core desire to fuel your goal, your subconscious mind will be working against you, sabotaging your conscious efforts instead of fueling and supporting them. And as I've said, when it comes to a contest between the conscious and the subconscious, the subconscious will win every time.

No doubt this is exactly what you've experienced in the past. But don't get me wrong—I'm not criticizing you for having failed to achieve your goals. I'm just trying to make you understand why you have failed so that it won't happen again.

Now that you've determined your behaviors and goals, it's time to get to the heart of the matter—identifying and connecting with your true core desire.

Step Three: Think About How You'll Feel Once Your Goals Are Achieved

The first question I ask my clients at Miraval is, "In the past, what is it you wanted to achieve by going to the gym and/or hiring a personal coach or trainer?" More than 80 percent of the time, I get the same answers: "I wanted to lose weight" or "I wanted to be fit and to feel better." But there is never any real excitement in their voices as they give those answers. It is only when I redirect my clients through deep listening and genuine inquiry (which is what I'm asking you to do for yourself here) that they are able to connect their goals to a true core desire, and when they do, their answers are suddenly full of passion: "I want to lose weight because I'm tired of being tired" or "I want to feel energized and alive again." Do you hear the difference? Can you feel the sense of excitement in that second set of answers?

A true core desire is much more than a reason. All of us have many reasons for doing many things, and we can probably think of just as many reasons for *not* doing those same things. A reason, therefore, can be nothing more than an excuse.

- *I'm going to go to the gym even though I have a lot of work to do because I really want to get fit and look good in my clothes. I'll make time to get my work done later.* That's a reason to go to the gym.
- *I'm not going to go to the gym even though I want to get fit and look good in my clothes because I have too much work to do and I don't have the time.* That's an equally valid reason *not* to go to the gym.

How often have you come up with similar "reasons" for doing or not doing something?

A reason is intellectually based; it comes from your conscious mind. A true core desire is a reason that comes from deep within your subconscious, and once you have identified it, it will release a positive, magical feeling that will enable you to fulfill your goal however many obstacles you face. This step, therefore, is the key to discovering and connecting with your true core desire.

For each of the goals you identified in step 2, ask yourself a question such as the following:

- *How will I feel when I am _____?* (twenty pounds lighter; fit and healthy; able to run a mile without stopping; not so stressed all the time—whatever your particular goals might be)
- *How will I feel when I have _____?* (lost those twenty pounds I haven't been able to get rid of; developed the stamina to play a game of hoops with my kids; managed to get my cholesterol down—whatever your own goals might be)

Visualize yourself having achieved the goal, listen to your inner voice, and feel the emotion attached to your answer. Remember to focus on the seeing, feeling, and being upon reaching your goal. Avoid thinking about what it will take to get there. Is your heart pounding with excitement? Does it feel great? Are you feeling anxious? Are you feeling fearful?

Now rate your sense of excitement on a scale of 1 to 10.

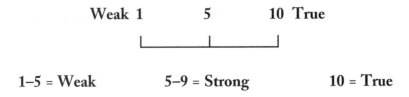

If your feelings are in the range of 1 to 5, they're pretty weak. Let's say that when you thought about how you'd feel when you fit into your size 6 jeans, you imagined that you would feel proud. But when you rated that feeling on the excitement scale, you gave it only a 5. Maybe what you would really like is to feel proud of yourself, and achieving that goal isn't so dependent on fitting into those jeans. That doesn't mean fitting into a pair of jeans isn't a perfectly valid goal, and you may well achieve it, but it's not possible to focus on more than one goal at a time, and what you're looking for here is a goal that's inspired by a true core desire.

Think of your goals as little mountains you are committed to climbing. When you reach the top of one, relax and celebrate, then start climbing the next and the next, until you don't feel a true core desire to climb any more mountains. In my opinion, that doesn't happen until we leave this world. Life is a series of mountains we climb, a series of celebrations we enjoy, and a series of new starts to which we look forward.

Let's move on. How would you feel if you got your cholesterol down? You'd be in control of your life; you could climb tall mountains. In fact, there would be nothing you couldn't achieve. Can you feel the joy? That's a 10!

A true core desire might make you feel:

- Excited
- Inspired
- Committed (You'll do anything it takes.)
- Grateful
- Comfortable
- Thankful

By contrast, when your goal does not represent a true core desire, you might feel:

- Confused
- Afraid
- Frustrated
- Uncomfortable
- Discouraged
- Angry

Once you've identified and connected with a true core desire, the magic within you will be released. That is a given because the magic flows from the desire. If you don't feel the magic, you can be pretty sure you haven't identified a true core desire.

Determine Your Level of Desire

Whenever you think about what you desire, you need to listen to your heart, because your desires emanate from your heart, not your head.

To determine the intensity of your desire, focus on the end result or outcome of achieving your goal. When a desire measures a 10 on the excitement scale, you'll feel true exhilaration. If you want to know what that feels like, focus on some event or occasion in the past that was exciting and exhilarating for you, something you achieved that really got your juices flowing. Remember what that felt like, and you'll know how it feels to connect with a core desire.

At the same time, when you feel that kind of excitement, your heart rate will automatically increase. To find your resting heart rate (RHR), which is normally between 58 and 72 beats per minute, place two fingers (not your thumb, which has a pulse of its own) on the pulse next to the indentation at the base of your neck or on the inside of your wrist. Find a clock or a watch with a second hand and count the number of heartbeats you feel in 15 seconds. Multiply that number by 4, and you have your RHR. Once you know that number, you'll be able to determine when your heart is beating faster because you've focused on what you truly desire.

If your heart rate doesn't go up when you concentrate on how you'll feel when you accomplish a particular goal, you can be fairly certain that you haven't identified a true core desire. Here's why.

There are both intrinsic and extrinsic factors involved in controlling your heart rate. Intrinsic regulation is what your body does every second of every day of your life to keep itself running smoothly. Extrinsic factors cause your heart rate to change rapidly because of a change in the chemicals that circulate in your blood or as a result of a direct command from your nervous system.

Extrinsic control is what occurs when you're watching a violent or romantic movie. You will be either anxious or excited, and your heart rate will increase. If you concentrate on something negative (something you don't want), the anxiety attached to that thought will cause your heart rate to increase. That's why it is necessary to focus on what you want rather than what you don't want when you go through this exercise.

If you concentrate on something you don't want, the increase in your heart rate may cause you to mistake fear for elation. What's worse, you'll be empowering your subconscious to send negative messages to your body. And as we've already discovered, when your subconscious speaks, your body has no choice but to listen.

If there is no change in your heart rate, you can be certain there is no emotion attached to your goal, which means that you're unlikely to continue pursuing it when the going gets tough. You may be interested, but you're not committed—you won't be willing to do whatever it takes.

A Word About Anxiety

In *The Power of Now*, Eckhart Tolle writes, "Fear resides either in the past or in the future; it cannot reside in the present." Feelings of anxiety can prevent you from recognizing a true core desire, even when you've identified it. If you do feel anxiety after identifying what you believe to be a true core desire, it may be because you're thinking about all the work you'll need to do to achieve your desire, and you're afraid of failing. That's why it's so important that you focus on how you'll feel when you achieve your goal, not on the process of attaining it.

Let's say, for example, that your goal is to climb to the top of a mountain. What you need to do is think about how you'll feel when you reach the peak. You'll be thrilled to see the world spread out around you. You'll be elated to have reached so high. You'll be feeling that if you did this, there's nothing in life you won't be able to achieve. But what if all you think about is how hard it will be to complete the climb? What if you keep imagining what might happen if you fell? What if you picture yourself stranded up there with no way to get back down? How do you think those thoughts would make you feel?

When you focus on the work rather than the fulfillment, the portion of your brain called the amygdala, which is involved in generating emotions, will release neurotransmitters that cause you to become anxious, and your anxiety will cause you to retreat back into your previous comfort zone. In the chapters that follow, I will supply you with a variety of tools to help you reconnect with your true core desire at times when you begin to feel anxious or frustrated. But just knowing about this aspect of your brain chemistry can save you from inadvertently denying yourself the right to succeed in achieving the positive outcome that will change your life for the better.

Moving from the Knowing to the Doing

According to Denis Waitley, author of *The Psychology of Winning*, "Procrastination is the fear of success. People procrastinate because they are afraid of the success that they know will result if they move ahead now." I've said that just by discovering and connecting with your true core desire, you'll release the inner magic that will guarantee your success. But that doesn't mean you can sit back and wait for the magic to begin. There is work to be done, and the next step in the process is to learn a few important techniques that will get you moving toward that core desire. If you're like most people, this will require shifting the negative thoughts you've been harboring about yourself and your ability to change so that you can begin to apply the power of your intention.

Before you take that step, however, you need to be totally committed to the process. So right now I'm going to ask you to sign the following simple contract with yourself. This voluntary agreement signifies your commitment to move forward.

VOLUNTARY AGREEMENT WITH MYSELF

Date: _____

I, the undersigned, commit and agree to furnish all the time and effort necessary to identify and connect with my true core desire.

I hereby commit to doing whatever it takes without being harmful to my health to achieve the optimal mental and physical performance I know is within me.

I will go the extra mile that is necessary to reach my goals because I know that not fulfilling my true core desire will only rob me of my right to be healthy, happy, and strong.

I understand that this is a process and that every step I take will bring me one step closer to my true core desire.

I have the power, I have the knowledge, I have what it takes, and I won't settle for anything less than my true core desire.

_____

Signature of Commitment

Two

Use the Power of Intention

The power of intention is your life force. It is what connects you to your higher self.

Dennis was one of the saddest, most out-of-shape people I'd ever met. His job was relentlessly demanding, and he didn't really enjoy the work he did. He had just come through an ugly, adversarial divorce, and he was in a precarious financial state. He'd been living with so much stress for so long that his overloaded brain was constantly releasing cortisol, the stress hormone, into his system. In essence, his body was in a perpetual state of "fight or flight"—a permanent panic—and the creative part of his mind had literally shut down as he retreated into his emotional safety zone. Now, in his mid-fifties, Dennis was not only flabby around the middle, with no muscle tone to speak of, but his spirit also had sagged to the point where, as he told me, he felt completely worthless as a human being.

I sat down with Dennis, as I do with all my clients, to ask the questions that would put him in touch with his true core desire—the very same questions I asked you in the previous chapter. He honestly assessed his current level of fitness and health as well as his level of stress. He thought about how he felt about his current state of health and well-being and what he would like to change. He then looked within himself to find the core desire that would truly motivate him to turn his life around once and for all. As he did these exercises, it became clear to Dennis that he was sick and tired of feeling sick and tired, and his deep, burning wish—his core desire—was to regain the sense of self-worth he'd had before the stresses of his job, his divorce, and his financial problems dragged him into such a negative pattern of feeling and doing.

At that point, I helped him to understand that everything he needed to make the changes he so deeply desired was already within him, and that his impetus to change would be fueled by the power of his intention.

At first Dennis was a bit puzzled and apprehensive. He didn't really understand what I meant by using the power of his intention. I then explained to him that if you value yourself as a caring and gentle person, yet find yourself sitting behind the wheel of your car screaming your head off at someone who has cut you off on the road, in that moment you're certainly not being the caring, gentle person you value. Similarly, if your intention is to be healthy, lose weight, and be full of energy, but your behavior shows that you are not exercising and are constantly eating unhealthy foods, you are not being true to what you value in and want for yourself.

The power of your intention is what allows you to match your behavior with what you truly want. Becoming mindful of your thoughts concerning your mental, physical, and emotional well-being is the first step toward getting in touch with that power. Like Dennis, you took that first step when you answered the questions about your health, fitness, and stress in the previous chapter. The second step was to focus on and define your goals, and the third was to look inward until you discovered the core desire that would provide the impetus for you to achieve whatever you want most for yourself.

In this chapter, I'll explain, as I did to Dennis, why you may still find it difficult to make your desire a reality, and I'll give you three of the most powerful tools I know of—meditation, visualization, and affirmation—to overcome those difficulties and fuel the positive inner power of your intention. That power is what will lead to your taking positive actions to make your desire a reality.

On an intellectual level, Dennis "got it"—he knew what he wanted, and he knew what he had to do to get it. On a deeper, emotional level, however, he was still afraid.

What Are You Afraid Of?

I said in the previous chapter that we humans instinctively fear change. Even after you've identified your core desire, you may be overcome by the anxieties that undermine your ability to connect with that desire. These anxieties can dampen the excitement you should be experiencing when you contemplate achieving your goal. When that happens, you need to take a long, hard look at yourself and confront what you're afraid of losing.

Dennis was afraid of everything. He was afraid of losing his job, losing his wife, and losing his money. Without those things, Dennis, in his own mind, was worthless or, worse yet, would cease to exist. In effect, Dennis had lost his sense of self (and self-worth) because his definition of self was based on external criteria. Because of his constant fear and anxiety, his conscious mind was sending his subconscious a continuous stream of negative thoughts that were not only causing him undue stress but also forcing him to expend all his energy fighting his fears. He simply had no energy left to commit to a healthy life.

If you define yourself and your happiness in terms of anything in the external world that is beyond your control—be it material goods or other people's opinions—you will always be afraid of losing it. Happiness will always be elusive. There's nothing wrong with wanting external things, but if wanting them is what motivates your behavior, you'll always be looking outside yourself for reasons to change.

I said earlier that no one else can motivate you. You need to seek motivation within yourself, and that is certainly true when it comes to finding happiness and achieving your core desire. To do that, you need to shift your conscious thoughts so that you begin to feed your subconscious mind positive messages about yourself and the things that are really important to you. That is how you fuel the power of your intention so that you will manifest those internal values in your behavior.

So how does all this relate to your quest for achieving health and fitness? Your body is an expression of who you are and what you value. If you are like most of us, when you get up in the morning and head into the bathroom, you can't help looking in the mirror. What are your thoughts then? Are you satisfied with what you see, or would you like to lose a little of this or gain a little of that? It doesn't matter what you want; what matters is that you get to the core of your desire and define your value in terms of that desire.

Most people don't look in the mirror and assess what they see in terms of their health. They don't "see" health. What they see is how they look in comparison to other people and what other people think of them. In other words, they define themselves based on external factors. There is nothing wrong with being motivated by external factors such as looking good in your jeans (or looking better than your ex-husband's girlfriend) if that works for you. But if you shift your thoughts so that you also define your goal in terms of your own health and happiness—regaining control of your blood pressure, managing your stress, or running with your kids in the park—you will be getting in touch with the power of your intention as it relates to what you value and want for *yourself*, which will be much more likely to ensure that you achieve your goal.

By now you may be both nodding and shaking your head. Sure, you understand that you need to shift your focus, but you still don't know how to go about it. After all, if it were that easy, you'd have done it a long time ago, and you probably wouldn't be in the place you are now. I understand all that, but I also promise you that the techniques I'm about to provide have all the power you need to get you from knowing to doing.

It's Time to Change Your Subconscious Tapes

If you're overweight and out of shape and you're not happy about it, it's probably because, subconsciously, you're getting something out of eating and/or being sedentary that you're afraid to give up. Do you eat to comfort yourself? Is being fat a reason to avoid social situations that frighten you? Do you think you don't have time to exercise regularly? Are you embarrassed to go to the gym? By using the three powerful tools I'm about to provide—meditation, visualization, and affirmation—you can change those thoughts. You can change your subconscious choices. You can choose to be slim, fit, and happy, just as you've chosen to be overweight, out of shape, and unhappy.

There's an old Native American legend about the white wolf fighting the black wolf. If we equate the white wolf with positive energy and the black wolf with negative energy, which one do you think will win the fight? It's the one you feed the most—your choice!

Remember, you're already committed to doing whatever it takes. You've signed that letter of commitment to yourself. Now you need to stop feeding the black wolf and start feeding the white one by rerecording the negative tapes that have been playing in your subconscious and preventing you from finding the happiness you seek.

Think about this: the conscious mind is capable of processing 2,000 bits of information per second, while the subconscious mind can process 4 billion bits per second. Which do you think will help you to give up bad habits and begin to replace them with good ones?

The Amazing Power of Meditation

Meditation is a practice that allows you to relax your body and quiet your conscious mind. It is a way to *not* think. It is one of the most useful tools I know for tapping into the power of the subconscious. Practitioners of Eastern religions have long known this, of course, but recent technological advancements in neuroscience have actually been able to demonstrate visually the positive effects of meditation on the brain. Recently, Dr. Dharma Singh Khalsa, president and medical director of the Alzheimer's Prevention Foundation and author of *Brain Longevity*, completed a study using SPECT (single-photon emission computed tomography) to show the effects of meditation on the brain. In the SPECT images below, we can clearly see the increased blood flow to the brain that occurs after meditation.

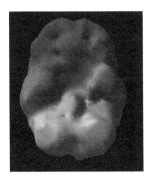

Before: This is a SPECT scan of the brain before meditation. The dimples in the front show a lack of complete blood flow. The area in the back region of the brain is lumpy and asymmetrical, also due to a lack of blood flow. In the center of the brain, no thalamus is detected. The thalamus controls appetite and sleep cycles, sets the emotional tone of the mind, and promotes bonding.

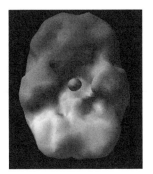

After: This SPECT scan shows the same brain after meditation. The dimples have disappeared, showing an increase in blood flow. The back of the brain is fuller and more symmetrical. The thalamus is now detected in the center of the brain.

In terms of health and fitness, meditation is the bridge that connects the body and mind. Meditation provides a razor-sharp sense of awareness that enables you to identify with the mental, physical, and emotional aspects of your being. By facilitating the amazing and extremely sophisticated relationship between your body and mind, you will be able to listen to the conversation that is taking place between the two, and when you do that, you will be mentally prepared to overcome any challenge you encounter in your quest for health and fitness.

If you've never tried meditation before, now is the time. I think you'll be amazed by how easily your stress melts away as the constant chatter of your conscious mind is silenced and the creative power of the subconscious takes over. Following are some of the many benefits to be reaped.

- Enhanced state of awareness
- Increased creativity
- Reduced stress
- Lower blood pressure
- Reduced anxiety
- Elevated mood
- Increased ability to focus

If you've never meditated before, you may feel a bit uncomfortable in the beginning. Don't worry about that. The more you practice, the more comfortable you'll feel. And don't be concerned if you have a hard time "clearing your mind." Thoughts will intrude, and that's okay. Just accept them and go back to your breathing. You can also use a *mantra,* a word such as *one* or the name of a loved one, to help you focus.

There are four simple requirements for practicing meditation.

- A comfortable position
- A quiet environment
- A mental device (such as your mantra)
- A focused attitude

MEDITATION FOR MENTAL GROUNDING

1. Give yourself permission to stop whatever you're doing and take ten to twenty minutes to be alone in a place where you won't be disturbed. Tell yourself that this time is for your well-being and that you have the right to take it for yourself. You will become more effective and energized if you think of it as your "sacred time alone." I have found that the best time to meditate is right after your morning shower, before you get dressed for the day. If that time isn't possible for you, just pick one that is.

2. Relax your body by doing some yoga or doing the deep-breathing exercise described on page 19. If you're not doing this right after your shower, you might want to relax by taking a hot bath. Lighting incense also will help because inhaling the scent will signal neurotransmitters in your brain to produce hormones that calm and soothe the mind. Find a quiet spot where you will not be disturbed, and sit comfortably in a chair or on the floor with your legs crossed in front of you. It is better not to lie down because you don't want to fall asleep during meditation. It may also be helpful if you choose an object to focus on to improve your concentration.

3. Pick any word, sound, short prayer, or phrase on which to focus. Some examples are *peace, love, blue, heal,* or simply *one.* Close your eyes, and as other thoughts come into your mind (and they will), just let them go and return to your focus word. You can say, "Oh, well, (your name), relax, one." Each time you inhale, imagine that you are breathing in an abundance of health. With each exhalation, breathe out the stress and begin to relax every muscle in your body, starting with your feet. Once you feel your feet relax, move on to your ankles, then your calf muscles, and so on, all the way up to your head. Feel your body getting lighter and lighter until you feel yourself floating. Empty your mind of all thoughts and concentrate on floating on a soft cloud.

4. When you feel the time has passed, simply open your eyes and check your watch or clock (no alarms, please). If the time isn't up, repeat the process until it is. Then take a deep breath, stretch upward, and relax your arms down.

The stress reduction created by meditation will bring you not only a deep sense of physical relaxation but also a new level of mental clarity. I'm sure you're aware of how stress can make you feel as if you're physically tied up in knots and your brain is so overloaded that you can't think clearly. But did you know that it can also contribute to your remaining overweight? That's one more reason for using the power of meditation to reduce your stress level.

When you are under stress, your brain produces a chemical that signals your adrenal gland to release a series of hormones, one of which is cortisol. When you are under constant stress, you are living with chronically high levels of cortisol, which, studies have shown, leads to increased storage of belly fat. Cortisol mobilizes fuel stored in the body as fat and glucose for quick action so that you can get out of whatever situation is causing your stress. That worked great for our ancestors, whose stressful situations usually involved some kind of physical danger that required them to fight back or flee. But when you can't do anything to escape the stress, because its cause is mental and emotional rather than physical, all that extra fuel goes unused and is simply re-stored as more fat.

So it's important to reduce stress not only to clear your mind for positive, creative endeavors but also to reduce the increased cortisol levels that are almost surely contributing to keeping you fat.

I worked with Dennis to help him learn meditation techniques so that he would be able to reduce the stress caused by external circumstances and refocus his energy in positive ways. Physically, this helped reduce the elevated cortisol levels that had been keeping him overweight. Mentally, the shift in his energy and attention allowed him to refocus the power of his intention so that he could create the happiness and success he desired.

Visualization: Using the Movie Screen of Your Mind

Sports psychologists are well aware of how athletes use visualization to enhance their performance and help ensure their success. Studies have shown that athletes who "practice" their sports mentally by visualizing themselves hitting a hole in one or breaking the tape to win a race improve their performance just as much as those who practice physically. And the more detail they are able to "see" in their minds, the more effective the visualization will be. For example, American swimmer Megan Quann, who defeated the reigning champion, Penny Heyns of South Africa, in the 100-meter breaststroke at the Sydney Olympics in 2000, took a stopwatch to bed every night before the event and visualized her race stroke by stroke. She said that in her visualization, she could see the tiles at the bottom of the pool, hear the crowd cheering, and actually taste the water. Similarly, the great basketball player Bill Russell describes a visualization he did as an eighteen-year-old watching a high school game from the bench. He was studying the moves of one of the most successful players on the team, Eural McKelvey, who went on to play for the Harlem Globetrotters. "Since I had an accurate vision of his technique in my head, I started playing with the image . . . running back the pictures several times and each time inserting a part of me for McKelvey. . . . When I went into the game, I grabbed an offensive rebound and put it in the basket just the way McKelvey did. It seemed natural, almost as if I were stepping into a film and following the signs."

When I was training for bodybuilding competitions, I used to visualize each part of my body going through my workout routine, seeing my muscles as full and symmetrical and my form as precise and perfect. Visualizing my workouts before I did them allowed me to imprint these images on my subconscious so that my body would seek to fulfill what I had created in my mind.

Visualization is really nothing more than using your inner eye to project an image or a series of images on the movie screen of your mind. What you can see on the screen of your mind, you can have in the movie of your life.

When we see something in the world around us, that image is sent to and stored in the brain. The mental images we create for ourselves are stored in the same way. The brain doesn't differentiate between what we see in actuality and what we see in our imagination. The old adage "Seeing is believing" holds just as true for mental "seeing" as it does for seeing with our eyes. Whatever outcomes we visualize for ourselves are imprinted on the brain as occurring in actuality. What this means is that we are able to manifest our own destiny.

When one of my clients has a problem visualizing what it would be like to achieve her goal, I tell her to find a picture in a magazine that shows the body she wants to attain (I also remind her to be sure that the picture she chooses is realistic for her), cut the head off the body, and replace it with a picture of herself. Then I tell my client to focus on that picture and study it every morning and every evening before she goes to sleep. When the client does that, it helps her to "see" what she's been unable to visualize in her mind.

If you are finding it difficult to visualize yourself at your goal weight, for example, try this approach. It worked for me. When I was beginning my career, I cut out pictures of two Mr. Universes from bodybuilding magazines and hung them on the wall in my room. Without even realizing it at the time, I was visualizing myself as having a body like theirs, and within a few years I was competing against those very same guys! I now have what I call a visualization board in my office on which I put pictures of the things I want to attain and the accomplishments I want to achieve.

Take a few minutes at the beginning of each day to visualize yourself completing the tasks you have set for yourself—going to the gym and working out, eating in accordance with your diet plan—and then seeing on the screen of your mind how you will do these things and how you will look and feel when you've accomplished them. If you do, you'll find that your brain will use these imprinted images to make your reality match what you've achieved in your imagination.

VISUALIZE YOUR VICTORY

Close your eyes and visualize yourself achieving your true core desire. Make the picture as detailed and vivid as you possibly can. What do you look like? How does it feel? Can you smell it, even taste it? The more vivid you're able to make your visualization, the more powerful it will be.

It may take a while for you to feel completely comfortable doing this. At first the images may not be entirely clear. That's okay, because the more you practice, the clearer the images will become. Try to picture the same things every day, adding more detail as you become more familiar with the process. Think of yourself as the lead actor in a movie you are projecting on the screen of your mind. Make sure that when you are doing this, you give an Oscar-winning performance.

Affirmation: Using Positive Self-Talk

In the previous chapter, I talked about the fact that my client Beth had been telling herself she was fat for so long that her body had no choice but to follow the dictates of her mind. I'm sure that many of you are using the power of your mind to undermine your body in much the same way. How often do you tell yourself "I'm tired," "I'm angry," or "I'm stressed-out"? What effect do you think those negative statements are having on your weight-loss and fitness efforts?

Another client, Michelle, lost more than eighty pounds in eight months. At one point, she was afraid of backsliding and called me to help her. When I asked how she was doing, she replied, "Great! I'm keeping the weight off, but it's a constant daily battle."

That "but" was a dead giveaway for me. If that's how she was responding to everyone who asked how she was doing, she was affirming that maintaining her weight loss was a "constant daily battle," and sooner or later those words would manifest themselves in her giving up the battle.

I reminded Michelle that she needed to be mindful of what she affirmed to herself and to others and suggested that instead of saying her fitness regimen was a constant battle, she say, "I am overcoming daily challenges." You can see how simply changing that statement allowed her to go from a negative to a positive attitude toward achieving her desire to maintain her new weight.

Here are a few simple rules to remember when you're creating positive affirmations for yourself.

- Always use the present tense. You want your mind to know that what you affirm has already happened.
- Be absolutely positive. Use as many positive verbs as you can.
- Be emotionally involved with your affirmations.
- Write them down so that you will remember them. Keep them short and specific.
- Personalize them by using your name.
- Repeat them as often as possible to imprint what you are affirming on your subconscious mind.
- Create a habit by setting aside a specific time for doing your affirmations each day.
- Believe that what you say is actually happening. The more you are able to believe, the stronger your affirmation will be.

100 AFFIRMATIONS
FOR THE BODY, MIND, AND SPIRIT

I have found these affirmations to be particularly powerful for many people, including myself. Read through them and use whichever ones speak most directly to you. Or use them as a template or inspiration for creating your own unique affirmations. Don't forget to affirm all aspects of your being—body, mind, and spirit.

Repeat each affirmation three times with feeling, and trust that with practice everything in your life will gently fall into place for your highest good. Take a minute to let go of all your limitations and allow your heart's desires to be created.

Affirmations for the Body

1. I have the power to control my health.
2. I deserve to be fit now.
3. I am ready, willing, and deserving to be fit.
4. I adopt healthy behaviors.
5. I focus on my form while I exercise.
6. I respect and appreciate others who are fit.
7. I am guided by my true core desire.
8. I am strong, lean, and beautiful.
9. I am losing the unwanted weight surely and smoothly.

10. I am strong, intelligent, and handsome.

11. I am in control of my health and wellness.

12. I have abundant energy, vitality, and well-being.

13. Health and vitality flow into my veins.

14. I am healthy in all aspects of my being.

15. I am maintaining my ideal weight.

16. I am burning fat easily.

17. I am fit, healthy, and happy.

18. I am full of energy to do all my daily activities.

19. I feel all the nutrients flowing into my cells.

20. I avoid junk food.

21. I am free of bodily pain when I work out.

22. I am burning fat and toning my body.

23. I feel sickness disappear from my body when I work out.

24. I ease my mind and work my body.

25. I visualize every muscle cell during my workout sessions.

26. I love and care for my body, and it cares for me.

27. I eat good, healthy foods.

28. I exercise regularly and feel great afterward.

29. I look and feel the best I have ever been.

30. I love the feeling of being fit.

31. I love the freedom of being healthy and fit.

32. I am in perfect health for as long as I truly desire.

33. I lead my family to the path of health and wellness.

34. I have physical strength and attractiveness for as long as I truly desire.

35. I am responsible for scheduling my time for exercise in advance.

36. I am comfortable with having a beautiful body.

37. My passion for health and wellness inspires others.

38. I love getting my workouts done.

39. I see myself having a beautiful body.

Affirmations for the Mind

40. I am in control of my stress levels.

41. I am canceling all negative thoughts and replacing them with new, positive ones.

42. I relax my body and work my mind.

43. I keep appointments with myself.

44. My mind and soul are at peace.

45. I always maintain the power to be positive.

46. I have total freedom to do whatever I truly desire.

47. I am persistent in my thoughts and actions.

48. The power of my persistence generates growth.

49. I have real personal confidence and a very positive self-image.

50. I now succeed effortlessly.

51. With laser-sharp focus, I prioritize my time and resources.

52. I make the time to exercise.

53. I am in control of my ego.

54. I am focused on the present moment.

55. I am calm and at peace with my challenges.

56. I am letting go of my negative thoughts.

57. I am worthy of a sharp and intelligent mind.

58. I am intelligent and charming, and I love being that way.

59. It's easy for me to accomplish my goals.

60. I am excited and passionate about my true core desire.

61. I am excited and passionate about achieving my goals.

62. I celebrate my life today and every day.

63. My enthusiasm about my goals helps me achieve them easily.

Affirmations for the Spirit

64. My mind and spirit are at peace.

65. The universe is open to me.

66. My love of life is rewarded.

67. I trust the universe.

68. I am an inspiration to others.

69. I am one with my spirit, body, and mind.

70. I am free to be myself.

71. I am a role model to my children.

72. I am a role model to my family.

73. I am a forgiving and loving person.

74. I have given myself permission to be at one with the universe.

75. I am worthy of love.

76. I am in touch with my feelings.

77. The more love I give, the more love I get.

78. The more I give, the more I receive.

79. I am grateful for everything I have and all the people I know.

80. The highest self within me now manifests perfect health in all my being and body.

81. I am responsible for my life and take charge of it.

82. I am at peace with the universe.

83. I love and accept myself.

84. I am a unique and loving person.

85. I am safe and always feel protected.

86. I create lasting friendships.

87. I acknowledge all my feelings.

88. I am surrounded with loving, caring people.

89. I am loving and accepting of others.

90. I trust my inner being to lead me on the right path.

91. I do all I can every day to create a loving environment for all, including myself.

92. My inner vision is always clear and focused.

93. I am committed to whatever I truly desire.

94. I now create inner peace and transformation.

95. I am an open channel for endless creativity.

96. I am connected deeply and intimately with my higher self.

97. It is natural to be happy.

98. My connection with infinite intelligence is now easily yielding the achievement of my true core desire.

99. I respect and help others who need my experience, knowledge, and skills.

100. I trust the universe and know that it works perfectly.

Write down your affirmations and post them prominently in your home and your office, even in your car. Just looking at your affirmations will be a constant reminder of your new beliefs about yourself.

Using affirmations is a powerful way for you to feed the white wolf instead of the black one. Think how much energy you've subconsciously been expending to record the negative tapes that have been keeping you stuck in negative behaviors. Now's the time to use the positive power of your intention to purposefully redirect that energy and record new, positive tapes. If the subconscious choices you've been making can have so much power over you, think how much more powerful your conscious choices can be.

Combining Your Tools to Increase Their Power

By using the techniques in this chapter, Dennis was able to harness the power of his intention to achieve his true core desire. He went from being a man who was flabby in body, mind, and spirit to being one who absolutely knew there was nothing he desired that he couldn't achieve. He lost fifty pounds in six months and told me he was feeling so good about himself that he was even considering competing as a senior bodybuilder!

Meditation, visualization, and affirmation are all tools that will help you create a harmonious relationship among your body, mind, and spirit so that all of your being is working together rather than pulling you in different directions—whether you're aware of it or not.

I have found that if you practice them all together, one following directly upon the other, at a particular time of day, their power will be exponentially increased. Therefore, I would urge you to set aside the necessary time for doing this. Ideally, it would be in the morning—when you are less likely to be distracted and more likely, shortly after awaking, to be in touch with your inner self—so that you will be starting your day with your mind already primed to manifest what you most want to create in your life.

Putting Your Intention into Action

You now know what you truly desire, and you have the tools you need to fuel the power of your intention to achieve it. What you need next is a viable plan of action. If you remember my story, my original plan—to join the gymnastics team—wasn't appropriate or viable because I hadn't yet developed the muscle strength I needed to perform. Instead, I had to take intermediate steps that would get me from being a 108-pound weakling to having the power to perform that iron cross on the still rings. I could visualize it all I wanted, but until I took the practical steps necessary to achieve my vision, it just wasn't going to happen.

In the following chapter, I'll give you all the information and tools you need to make sure the plan you create for achieving your core desire is the one that's going to get you to your goal.

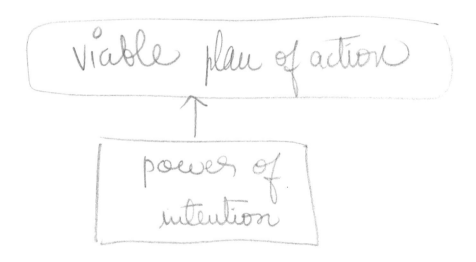

Three

Make an Appropriate Action Plan

No valid plans for the future can be made by those who have
no capacity for living now.
—Alan W. Watts, *The Wisdom of Insecurity*

Meet Mike, an intern at a big-city hospital who was caught in a vicious cycle. Mike spent long, stressful hours at the hospital every day, and when he was on call, even his short periods of sleep might be interrupted over and over again. He was also overweight, out of shape, and eating a very poor diet on the run. His super-busy schedule was interfering with his ability to take care of his health, and his poor health was making it even more difficult for him to cope with the stresses of his career. He needed to get off this self-destructive merry-go-round, but he couldn't figure out how to do it. That's when he came to see me.

As we talked, Mike filled me in on a bit of his personal history. As it turned out, he was the son of a physician who had let his family know that he expected them to be exactly like him—that is, smart, successful, and in great physical shape. According to Mike, both his siblings seemed to have fulfilled those expectations without any difficulty, while only he had struggled. In essence, he believed that he deserved to be fat and unloved. He'd gone to medical school as a way to regain the love and respect of his father. He also had a history of taking speed and other drugs to lose weight. As an intern, he had easy access to these dangerous medications, and it had taken a trip to the emergency room to make him realize that he desperately needed to make some changes in his life.

As we talked, I was able to show Mike that it wasn't really his busy schedule that was preventing him from taking care of himself. Rather it was the negative subconscious messages that were telling him he deserved to be overweight and was unworthy of his father's love. We talked about the fact that he couldn't base his happiness on what his father wanted for him, and that he needed to reframe his weight-loss goals to reflect what he truly desired for himself.

Once he had embraced his core desire to become a fit and healthy role model for his patients and had released the power of his intention by visualizing and affirming that goal to himself, we were able to come up with a plan for him to include exercise and healthy eating in his daily schedule. Now, as a practicing physician, he is lean and fit. When his patients claim they don't have time to do what it takes to ensure their own fitness, he tells them his own story as a way to inspire, motivate, and encourage them.

The Power of a Plan

You may not be an overworked intern, but we all have a hard time putting our good intentions into action. You may be an overstressed workaholic who can't find the time to prepare healthy meals. Or an overscheduled soccer mom ferrying three kids to school, playdates, and doctor's appointments. Maybe you're a member of the "sandwich generation," working full-time, raising kids, and taking care of aging parents. All of those are real obligations. But I guarantee that by making an appropriate action plan that is fueled by the power of your intention, you *will* be able to find time for fitness and achieve your core desire.

Tai, a Vietnamese American I met recently, is a perfect example of someone who needed a potentially life-threatening wake-up call to rediscover the balance he'd somehow lost along the way. Tai had been raised to believe that America was the land of opportunity. Even before coming to this country twenty-six years ago, his core desire was to start his own business. He was convinced that he would succeed because that's what he'd been taught, and with time he manifested what he believed.

His initial plan for achieving his desire was not, however, what I would call a healthy one. To achieve the American dream, Tai believed that he needed to work sixteen hours a day and become as stressed-out as all the Americans he saw around him. He became so caught up in the rat race that he even stopped practicing the meditation he had learned in Vietnam.

Unfortunately for Tai, he not only built a small business empire for himself, but he also built a serious health disaster waiting to happen. One day, in the middle of a crowded store, he suffered a heart attack. At the age of forty-eight, he underwent heart bypass surgery. After he recovered, he resolved to eat a healthier diet and reschedule his time so that he could exercise daily and fit meditation back into his stress-filled life. Now, three years later, he is in good health, thanks to his decision to slow down and return to the healthy habits he had lost along the way—mediating, exercising, and eating right. "I can't believe that I fell right into that trap, thinking that by abusing myself I'd be happy," Tai told me. "If I died, what then? Who would take care of my kids? The business can always take care of itself."

Like Tai, I lost track of my core desire when, as a successful bodybuilder, I began to focus solely on my body and was driven by the fear of losing a competition. At that point, my plan no longer included nourishing my mind and spirit, and instead of being happy, I was once again anxious and miserable. If your "plan" is simply to amass wealth and possessions or to receive recognition from others—if it doesn't include time to nourish your mind and spirit—you, like Tai and me, will need to adjust it so that it honors and balances the three basic expressions of life.

The Three Fundamental Expressions of Life

I believe that to live a truly meaningful life, we must learn to balance its three basic aspects—body, mind, and spirit—by honoring the importance of each one and setting goals for achieving each aspect's optimum expression. If you're familiar with traditional Chinese philosophy, you have heard about the ancient concept of balancing yin and yang—the two opposing forces found in all things in the universe—to optimize chi, or life force. Ayurveda, the traditional healing philosophy of India, is also based on finding a balance in your mental and emotional states and connecting with your spirit to heal your body.

My own philosophy of living a life in balance is based on the wisdom of the ancients as it is applied to the modern world. I don't believe that you have to reject material things to achieve mental and spiritual well-being, but I do believe that you need to find a balance among all three to feel good about yourself and find true happiness in all aspects of life. Look at the following list and let it guide you to consider where you might be able to shift a few priorities to find more balance and, as a result, more happiness and success—mentally, physically, and emotionally—in your life.

Body

- Breathing
- Hygiene
- Skin care
- Exercise
- Playing sports
- Sexual activity
- Nutrition
- Relaxation
- Positive speech
- Body posture
- Clothing
- Jewelry
- A comfortable home

Mind

- Creativity
- Work
- Entertainment
- Music
- Reading
- Traveling
- Education
- Meditation
- Reflection
- Visualization
- Affirmation
- Writing

Spirit

- Enlightenment
- Awareness
- Love
- Compassion
- Gratitude
- Forgiveness
- Generosity
- Altruism
- Friendliness

This list is not intended to be exhaustive or definitive. Not all of these items will be equally important to you, and maybe there are others you would add to your own inventory of things that would make you feel fulfilled in body, mind, and spirit. Remember that the key here is to find balance, and the following exercise is designed to help you do just that.

WHAT ARE YOU DOING WITH YOUR TIME?

We all schedule our time, at least to some extent. We may not actually write down our schedule, but we do have some idea how long it takes us to do all the things we need to accomplish every day. The questions included here are a way to help you schedule the time you have available, but they are meant to do more than that. By completing this exercise, you will be able to see what you really value in life and whether you've been directing your time and energy toward nurturing all aspects of yourself. Sadly, in today's society, many of us are so busy just getting things done that we neglect our bodies and fail to nurture our mental and spiritual well-being.

To help you see where you're directing your energy, complete the following schedule by filling in the amount of time you spend doing each activity each week. Then add up the total number of hours.

- Traveling to and from work:

- Working in the workplace:

- Working at home in the evening and/or on weekends:

- Talking on the phone to family and friends:

- Dating or socializing with friends:

- Spending time with family and/or caring for children:

- Doing chores and taking care of personal business:

- Sleeping:

- Eating:

- Exercising:

- Pursuing hobbies and other leisure activities, such as reading or watching TV:

- Pursuing spiritual activities, including meditation:

Total hours:

Now ask yourself the following questions.

1. Have you allowed enough time to do all the things you want or need to do? Remember that you *need* to spend time nurturing yourself and your loved ones. You *need* to devote time to *being* the person you want to be, not just *doing* the tasks you need to get done. *(Subtract your total hours from 168, the total number of hours in a week.)*

2. Have you allowed enough time for physical, mental, and emotional fitness? *(You should schedule at least 10 minutes of working both your mind and your body for every hour you are at work. So if you work 8 hours a day, you need to schedule 80 minutes for mental and physical fitness each day.)*

3. What can you do to adjust your schedule so that there will be enough time for everything you want or need to do? *(Go back to the first question and see which aspects of yourself you may have been shortchanging and how you can create a better balance in your life.)*

As I tell my clients, everything we have to do in life—except meditation and visualization—is a stressor (and that includes good things such as getting married and playing with our children), so you *do not* want to create additional stress by adding more time commitments to your life. Instead, you need to find ways to intelligently redistribute your time. In other words, try to determine how much time you spend doing things (such as working fifteen hours a day) that cause you *bad* stress. Then shift some of that time to something that causes you good stress (such as working out at the gym). For example, if you eat a big lunch in the office and then sit at your desk being unproductive for the next half hour because you've overstressed your body with too much food, try to use that unproductive time more productively by going to the gym (and eating a lighter meal). Think about redistributing your time the way you think about changing your diet. You don't change your diet by simply *adding* healthy foods to the unhealthy ones you're already eating. Doing that would be counterproductive. Instead, you *replace* unhealthy foods with healthy ones. You can apply the same principle to how you spend your time by replacing time used unproductively with time used to nurture your mental, emotional, and physical well-being.

Figuring out how to use your time more productively (making a realistic plan) may require some trial and error. Remember that if you are capable of honoring appointments with others, you are capable of honoring appointments with yourself.

Schedule your workout appointments at least thirty days in advance and post them where you'll be sure to see them every day—on the refrigerator door, for example, or on the bulletin board in your office. Make appointments with yourself for mental reconditioning (meditation, visualization, and affirmation) for the next three months. Write them in your daily calendar and do not cancel on yourself unless you absolutely have to. Doing this will be a powerful reminder that you are the only one responsible for achieving your true core desire. This is not being self-ish, because if you can't or don't take care of yourself, you will be that much less able to take care of your loved ones.

Find a Coach or Trainer Who Can Be a Mentor

This book provides all the information you need to achieve your health and fitness goals and can actually be used as your personal fitness coach. But one of the most common reasons for abandoning a fitness plan is frustration. If you don't know how to use gym equipment properly, you run the risk of either hurting yourself (worst-case scenario) or failing to see results (best-case scenario). For that reason, particularly if you have never used free weights or professional gym equipment before, I strongly recommend that you hire a competent personal trainer or fitness coach for at least a few weeks to show you how to use the equipment safely and to its best advantage. In addition, a coach or trainer can help keep you motivated during that initial period of four to six weeks until your routine becomes automatic.

It's true that no one can motivate or coerce you into achieving your goal. That motivation must come from within. But it's also true that virtually every successful person I've ever met, no matter what his or her field of endeavor, has said that he or she wouldn't have been able to do it all on his or her own. We all need to learn everything we can about whatever task we're about to undertake, and that often means asking for help from someone whom we can trust and who is an expert in his or her field.

Almost every gym has several trainers on staff who may differ in their methods, beliefs, and attitudes. You need to find the one who will be the best "fit" for you in terms of temperament, ideology, and personality. And if you don't find the right person at the first gym you go to, you need to look elsewhere. If you were buying a new pair of pants, you'd certainly try on several pairs until you found the one that fit you best. Finding a trainer to guide you through a fitness program is certainly a bigger, more important decision than buying a pair of pants. Here are some things to look for.

- **Experience.** I recommend no less than five years' experience working as a trainer or coach. There's nothing wrong with asking how long someone has been doing his job. If you were running a company and interviewing a potential new employee, you'd certainly ask that question. If you're paying your coach or trainer, he is your employee. That's something you need to remember.
- **Interpersonal skills.** Can you have a conversation with this person and convey what you want to get from the relationship? Is she responsive? Does she listen and try to accommodate your goals? Can she convey to you what she thinks you need to do in a way you understand? Lack of communication can undermine even your best, most strenuous efforts.
- **Education.** Again, if you were hiring an employee for your business, you'd want to know what education he has had in the area for which you are hiring him. Your potential coach or trainer should have completed training in kinesiology (the anatomy, physiology, and mechanics of body movement), anatomy, client assessment, program design, and basic nutrition. He also should have knowledge of human behavior in order to understand why a client who had been doing well might suddenly seem to lose motivation or fail to continue improving. In addition, he should hold current personal trainer or fitness coach certification from an accredited organization such as the American Council on Exercise, the American College of Sports Medicine, the National Academy

of Sports Medicine, or the National Strength and Conditioning Association, as well as a two-year degree in a related field, such as exercise science, exercise physiology, or physical education.

- **Punctuality.** Again, this is a quality you'd expect from any employee. If you've made time in your busy schedule to keep this fitness appointment with yourself, you have every right to expect that your trainer will honor that appointment with the same degree of punctuality.
- **Physical condition.** If your coach or trainer is overweight or out of shape, you ought to question how she can help you when she can't seem to take care of herself.
- **Physical hygiene.** This is another aspect of physical condition. Good hygiene is an expression of caring for one's body. If your trainer doesn't care for his own body, he probably won't be able to help you care for yours. In addition, working out in a gym is sweaty stuff, and you shouldn't have to be exposed to another person's sweat.

I would also recommend that the person you choose have knowledge of the mind-body connection and be familiar with meditation techniques as well as yoga, Pilates, tai chi, and other alternative health and fitness disciplines. Although this is certainly not mandatory, such knowledge is an indication that your trainer or coach is well-grounded and can increase the flow of positive energy during your training sessions.

Watch Out for Red Flags

Your coach or trainer should always behave professionally and appropriately. Here are some things to watch out for.

- Drinking, eating, or chewing gum while working with you. Doing these things is a sign of disrespect, and they could lead you to become sloppy yourself. Your trainer or coach ought to be your role model as well as your instructor.
- Appearing intoxicated or hungover.
- Dressing inappropriately. To me, a T-shirt and shorts or sweatpants are appropriate; a tank top and spandex pants are not. Again, it's a question

of showing you respect—as opposed to showing off his own personal equipment.

- Leaning on the equipment during training. If your trainer is lounging on the equipment, she is not engaged in the process or totally focused on you. She ought to be alert and ready to jump in and help you if you get into trouble on a piece of equipment.
- Taking time from your training to talk on the phone or greet or chat with other people. Remember, you've paid for this person's time and you deserve his full attention.
- Constantly looking at her watch. If she is so anxious for the session to be over, she's probably thinking about what she's going to do next and isn't fully present to you.
- Sticking with repetitive exercise programs that indicate a lack of innovation. If your trainer can't come up with a varied routine, he's probably bored—and pretty soon you'll be bored, too.
- Inappropriate physical contact. Your trainer needs to be watchful and alert and may need to touch you while spotting you on the equipment, but any further physical contact is crossing a personal boundary that may signal the crossing of other boundaries as well.
- Sharing personal problems. Like inappropriate physical contact, sharing personal problems is a sign that your coach does not understand or honor the professional nature of your relationship.
- Ignoring or dismissing your questions. You're the client, and your trainer should be courteous enough to respond. If she ignores or refuses to answer you, it may be because she doesn't have the knowledge to provide the information you need.
- Recommending supplements or herbs. That's the job of your physician.
- Diagnosing your injuries or illnesses. If you are ill or injured, your trainer should recommend that you see your doctor, not take on the role of diagnostician.
- Failing to return your phone calls or e-mails. When you're a professional in any field, you need to act like one—which means responding to messages left by phone or e-mail.

Beware of Client-Trainer Codependency

It always alarms me to hear from guests at Miraval that they have been working with a trainer for a year or more and have seen minimal or no results. Such situations signal what I call client-trainer codependency. The coach or trainer has become dependent on the client for income, and the client has become dependent on the coach or trainer to prevent him or her from failing (even though it ought to be perfectly clear that he or she has already failed).

I saw a shocking example of this when I met John, a regular client at Miraval. John was dropped by his trainer (who decided to go snowboarding) on one of his visits and was assigned to work with me instead. He told me that he'd been working with his trainer for ten years. When he began, he weighed more than four hundred pounds—and he still weighed more than four hundred pounds ten years later. His trainer had done nothing at all to help him change his life-threatening condition.

I conducted a general fitness assessment of John and then began working with him on the mental aspects of achieving his goal. At that time, John was so depressed that his only goal was to survive. The first thing he had to do was learn to believe in himself. Working with me, John lost three pounds in just three days, and that alone gave him hope that he could and would survive. Originally, his core desire was simply to make it through each day, but as he saw that he could lose weight, he began to desire a better life for himself. Looking at his goal from this new perspective was so powerful that he immediately felt a new surge of energy. I helped John to understand that he could use that newfound energy to fuel the positive power of his intention by visualizing himself when he'd lost more weight and regained his health and by affirming that he had the ability to do it. The belief that he actually could succeed left John in tears, and I was equally tearful to think of all the time and effort he'd wasted for so many years.

I believe that every trainer should be honest and honorable enough to understand that his clients are literally putting their lives in his hands, and if he is unable to help them achieve what he deems to be a reasonable degree of success, he ought to recommend that they find another trainer. But the client also needs to take responsibility. If, after four weeks, you are not seeing results and you have truly been following the program and doing what it takes to achieve your true core desire, you need to move on and find another coach. (As a rule of thumb, I would define "results" as losing at least one pound per week.)

Surround Yourself with People Who Support Your Efforts and Believe in Your Goal

A good coach or trainer may be your most important mentor, but other people in your life also can help to fuel your positive energy or to undermine your efforts to change your priorities and take care of yourself. Your spouse, your children, your parents, and your friends are all in some way involved in your quest for change. Although it's true that no one else is responsible for your failure to change, the encouragement and help of those closest to you can have a serious impact on your success.

Build a buddy system of family or friends who support you by letting you know whenever they notice a positive change. Let those close to you know that you're committed to achieving your core desire and that they can help you by affirming and acknowledging your progress.

Even better, ask someone who has similar goals to be your training partner. Look around when you're at the gym. Is there someone who seems to be similar to you in age and level of fitness and whose schedule coincides with yours? If so, perhaps you could team up with him or her to work out together. Just knowing that someone is counting on you to show up may provide the added incentive you need to stick to your program and may fuel your competitive spirit. But be prepared to go it alone if your partner slacks off or drops out.

Whenever possible, free yourself from "energy vampires"—unsupportive people in your life. If losing weight and becoming fit is your true core desire and the people with whom you surround yourself do not believe in your endeavor and are not themselves engaged in healthy habits, how can they *not* adversely affect your chances for success? I'm not suggesting that everyone around you has to be exercising and eating right (although that would be the ideal), but I am saying that they must at least help you by believing in you and supporting your efforts.

Amanda and Frank were living together when Amanda decided it was time to lose weight. After consulting with me, she made a tough decision. She realized that Frank was standing between her and her core desire. She knew that some things would have to change if they were to continue living together. Her argument was plain and simple: "How can I love someone who encourages me to stay eighty pounds overweight? What kind of love can I provide to Frank if I don't love myself? All we do is eat, go to the movies, or watch TV after work. What kind of life is that? Besides, Frank could really use new healthy behaviors, too. He'll thank me in the long run." Ultimately, Amanda determined that if Frank could not support her physically, mentally, and spiritually, they would have to separate.

Amanda and Frank decided that they both would follow the program, helping each other with motivation, inspiration, and, most important, love for the next three months. If, at the end of that time, they (and their relationship) were not feeling and looking better, they would reconsider their plan. By the end of that trial period, both had lost weight. They also felt great and realized that they loved each other more than either of them had realized.

I have worked with many couples, and I know that, almost invariably, if one of the partners is unhealthy and overweight, the other is in a similar condition. The same holds true for parents and children. Getting both partners or everyone in the family involved is absolutely critical for success.

Create a Positive Environment

You've been doing everything you can to erase negative messages from your subconscious and affirm your ability to achieve your true core desire. But if you see reminders of your past failures every time you look around, you'll be setting yourself up to respond to those external cues and return to your previous self-destructive habits. Remember that cues in your present experience can trigger the subconscious tapes that will cause you to revert to negative patterns. To make your external and internal environments reflect each other, try these strategies.

- Remember to set up your workout appointments thirty days in advance and make sure you have reminders clearly in view.
- Post your affirmations and your list of goals prominently in your home, your office, and your car.
- Put away all visual reminders—such as framed photographs—in which you appear unfit. Remember that these visual clues can trigger the subconscious tapes that will tell your body to remain overweight and unhealthy.
- As your body begins to change, take new pictures of yourself that act as external reminders of your new internal environment.
- Clean out the refrigerator and pantry and discard all the unhealthy food.

Believe me, everyone in your family, even your pet, will thank you for it in the long run.

- Keep healthy snacks—such as raisins, nuts, or cut-up vegetables—on hand at all times. Look at the food lists in chapter 5 for other healthy snack ideas.
- Make sure you have health magazines, books, and tapes around the house—even in the bathroom.
- Make use of mood-enhancing colors such as light green or sky blue (or whatever color makes you feel happy and upbeat). You can do this simply by using throw pillows and accessories or go all the way and repaint the walls. (Maybe you've been thinking about repainting anyway. If so, now is the time to do it.) Some of my clients even go so far as to create a mini-Miraval setting in their home with smooth stones and miniature cacti or ocotillo plants. They buy the candles we use in our classes or take home other souvenirs that remind them of the positive feelings they experienced at the spa. The point here is to create an environment that will give you positive feelings, however you choose to do it.
- Use a scented candle to give your home a fragrance that reminds you of a happy, fun time in your life. I use a lemon scent in my office because it reminds me of a special and wonderful time I once had traveling in Switzerland. Every time I smell the lemon, I remember that time, and that automatically lifts my mood.
- Record your affirmations and keep a CD or MP3 player near your bed so that you can listen to them just before retiring and immediately upon rising.
- To reduce stress, keep soothing and relaxing background music playing in your home and, if possible, in your office.
- Buy new clothing that is flattering and allows you to move. Buying new clothes that you intend to wear when you achieve your next goal can be a powerful motivational factor. When you reach that goal, don't be afraid to wear them. You deserve them!

You need to really think about what makes you feel good and gives you peace. It may be a color or an aroma. It may be something as simple as watching a movie that makes you laugh. Once you determine what those things are, you need to re-create that environment in your home, your office, and even your car—wherever you spend your time. If your environment is cluttered and chaotic, it will make you feel cluttered and chaotic as well. You need to create a peaceful space to create a peaceful life. Clear out the clutter, and you will be better able to clear and focus your mind.

I like to tell my clients the story of the man who went to his Zen master and said, "I'm going crazy in my house. I can't think straight." When the master asked him why that was, he said, "It's because I have a wife, eight kids, two sheep, four dogs, and three cats." So the master said, "Go home and every day kick one of them out." The man went home and did as the master told him, but when he'd kicked them all out, he felt sad. So he went back to the master and said, "I did as you told me, but now it's empty in my house, and I feel sad." The master told him, "Okay, now go home again and invite them back one by one until you feel happy; then stop." He missed his wife, so he invited her back. Then he invited each of his children. When he had them all back, he invited one dog and one cat. At that time, he was happy and no longer lonely, so he stopped.

I tell my clients to clear the clutter from their lives and replace what they've eliminated with things that make them happy.

Educate Yourself

Particularly if you are new to the idea of getting in touch with your spiritual self and harnessing the power of your mind to make the changes you want not only in your body but also in every aspect of your life, I would suggest that you seek out books and information on meditation, relaxation techniques, and other methods for connecting with your inner wisdom. Although this book provides all the basic tools you'll need to discover and connect with your true core desire so that you will be able to achieve your fitness and weight-loss goals, the more you learn, the better able you will be to put those tools to use and make them work for you.

One sure sign of achieving wisdom is understanding that there is always more to learn. I'm still learning, and I hope that I will never lose my desire to acquire new tools and to improve my skills. By reading or listening to tapes twenty minutes to one hour a day, I am constantly educating myself and learning new things so that I can help others even more. I've listed some of the books and tapes I've found particularly helpful in Further Resources (pages 183–186), but I encourage you to explore any others that will help you to better understand, connect with, and achieve your goal.

Be Ready to Make Adjustments

It's important to make a plan and put it into action, because every step you take will put you that much closer to achieving your true core desire. That said, you may need to adjust your initial plan, just as I did when I thought I could become a gymnast without first building muscle and stamina. You may be so excited to have discovered your core desire that you want to get there immediately. You need to be realistic. Either overestimating or underestimating your ability can be detrimental to achieving your goal. If you overestimate your ability, you may find that you can't live up to your plan. If you underestimate your ability, you may not see the results that keep you moving forward.

As you begin to take action on your own plan, you will experience many physical, mental, and emotional changes. Are you losing weight and feeling better? Do you feel more focused mentally and more at peace emotionally? You need to remain mindful and attentive to those changes, because they will let you know whether you need to make adjustments to your plan. What is working for you? What, if anything, is not? What can you do to put more emphasis on the positive and eliminate the negative as you go along?

As I've already mentioned, if you are feeling unhappy about any aspect of your life, it's because you've given yourself a reason to feel that way. *Only you can remove that reason.* When you have a need for something that is lacking in your life, you are out of balance, and you feel anxious because you are aware that you are missing something. When that happens, I suggest that you reevaluate your thoughts and feelings by going back over the various exercises in this book to help you discover the source of the imbalance.

What have you visualized for yourself? Are you acting in a way that reflects your new beliefs and values? Revisit the screen of your mind and consider whether you're doing the things that will get you where you want to go. If something in your life isn't working, you need to mentally retrace your steps to discover where you lost your way, exactly as you would if you'd lost some physical possession such as your car keys. If you lost your car keys, what would you do? You'd retrace your steps until you came to the place where you left them.

Here is an exercise that will quickly help you to figure that out where you stepped off the path and reconnect your behaviors with your goals.

MATCHING YOUR NEW BELIEFS WITH
YOUR BEHAVIORS

Sometimes you may drift from your plan because there is a conflict between your behaviors and your new beliefs—in other words, between your body and your mind. When that happens, you need to reconnect the two so that you can be true to yourself and your commitment to achieve your true core desire. This exercise will help you get back on track.

Write down your behaviors and match them with the new beliefs about yourself that you have created through meditation, visualization, and affirmation. Are they congruent or in conflict with one another?

Example:

I eat a Milky Way bar just before getting on the treadmill, and my new belief is to lose weight.

My behavior is _____.

My new belief is _____.

Does my behavior match my belief?

If you feel burned-out on your nutrition or exercise plan, you may simply be tired. Don't beat yourself up about it; just take a week off to relax.

If your strategy as a whole isn't working, the plan you came up with initially may not be appropriate for achieving your true core desire. But there are other possibilities as well. Maybe you simply doubt your ability to perform the tasks you have set for yourself, or you think it's too much work. If that's the case, remember that focusing on the outcome rather than the process is what will get you through.

Or perhaps you are continuing to feed the black wolf instead of the white wolf. A few years ago, I worked with a gentleman from Toronto who was doing just that. Although he is extremely handsome and very wealthy, my client couldn't seem to find his own happiness. After about a year, he called me to say, "Nordine, I still feel that I'm missing something in my life. I can buy and have anything I want. I'm in shape and I eat well, but every morning I wake up feeling anxious. What's wrong with me?"

"Nothing is wrong with you," I replied. "You've just forgotten about the many things you are grateful for. Write down twenty-five things you are grateful for and read them every morning."

Sometimes nothing is wrong with us; we just need to remember who we are and how wonderful our life is. So whenever you feel that you are not happy, I suggest that you do exactly what I recommended to my client: write down twenty-five things you are grateful for and focus on the positive instead of the negative. Doing this will not only make you feel better, but it will put you in a place of compassion for others who do not possess a fraction of what you have.

Following are twenty-five things for which I am grateful. When you're making up your own list, you may find that you're not able to stop at twenty-five. If so, let that be a sign and ask yourself, "Why in the world am I feeling so unhappy?"

1. I am grateful to have a new lease on life today.

2. I am grateful to have people who love me.

3. I am grateful to love.

4. I am grateful to have food on my plate.

5. I am grateful to have a home.

6. I am grateful for my health.

7. I am grateful to have an income.

8. I am grateful that I am able to exercise.

9. I am grateful to have friends.

10. I am grateful to have a family.

11. I am grateful to have work that I care about.

12. I am grateful for the ability to help others.

13. I am grateful to communicate with people around the world.

14. I am grateful for my freedom.

15. I am grateful for my education.

16. I am grateful for my pets.

17. I am grateful for my car.

18. I am grateful for my savings.

19. I am grateful for my accomplishments.

20. I am grateful to have good neighbors.

21. I am grateful to have intelligence.

22. I am grateful to have a healthy body.

23. I am grateful to be beautiful inside and out.

24. I am grateful for the clothes on my back.

25. I am grateful for my country.

What are you grateful for?

When You're Drifting Off Course, It's Time to Change Direction

Remember that when you have an appropriate action plan, you will be able to achieve your true core desire, no matter what challenges you encounter. Without a plan, you may follow the wrong path, which will prevent you from arriving at the place you want to be. So be honest and realistic about your abilities. Find a mentor, coach, or trainer to guide you. Surround yourself with supportive people whose goals are similar to your own. Keep reminders of your commitments and affirmations where you can see them every day. And be mindful of yourself so that you can make adjustments as needed. Just keep checking with yourself as if you were a sailor at the helm of a ship, and be willing and able to trim your sails or adjust your rudder accordingly.

The More You Do It, the Easier It Gets

Discovering your core desire will release the magic you have within to do whatever it takes to achieve your goal. But I'd be lying if I didn't also let you know that it will take determination and perseverance. At first you'll have to remain resolute in your commitment, but with time—and by that I mean no more than four to six weeks—your new habits and beliefs about yourself will be so internalized that they'll become automatic. In the next chapter, I'll tell you why that's so and how you can make sure that you continue to apply your resolve until it happens.

Four

Apply Your Resolve and Make It Automatic

As a single footstep will not make a path on the earth, so a single thought will not make a pathway in the mind. To make a deep physical path, we walk again and again. To make a deep mental path, we must think over and over the kind of thoughts we wish to dominate our lives.
—HENRY DAVID THOREAU

When Sarah walked into my office several years ago, I saw right away that she was quite beautiful. But at just over five feet tall and weighing well over two hundred pounds, she was also dangerously obese. As we began to talk, Sarah told me that she was forty-one years old, divorced, and looking for a new man in her life.

Before I answered her, I let Sarah know that she would probably be shocked and also offended by what I was about to tell her, but since she'd come to me for help, I assumed that she wanted me to be honest. I went on to say that it appeared to me she was actually trying to kill herself, and if she really wanted someone to love and care for her, she'd have to start loving and caring for herself first.

I know that my words were harsh, but I also know that it sometimes takes that kind of brutal honesty to help people shift their perspective and reframe their goals in terms of a true core desire. I was able to do that for Sarah by allowing her to understand that losing weight and becoming fit was not a goal to be sought in and of itself but rather a tool to help fulfill her desire to have a loving companion in her life.

If I'd left it there, however, I'd have been doing Sarah a great disservice, because I knew that making such a big change in her life would not be easy. Not only would she have to shift her mental attitude toward herself and her lifestyle, but she'd be facing significant physical challenges as well. So I made Sarah a promise: If she was willing to give me four to six weeks, I would stick with her, and she would be able to turn her life around. Armed with her newfound power of intention, Sarah agreed, and that very day we began to work together to develop an appropriate plan of action. We both knew that the plan could not be too ambitious because, at least in the beginning, doing any kind of physical exercise was going to be very difficult for her.

Only Four to Six Weeks?

At this point, I'm sure at least some of you are wondering how Sarah could possibly lose all the weight she needed to and get in shape in only four to six weeks. But that's not what I promised her. Go back and read it again. What I said was that I'd stick with her and that she would be able to turn her life around. She certainly wouldn't be able to reach her goal weight in those few weeks, but she *would* be able to rewrite the negative subconscious tapes that had been preventing her from doing what she truly desired. And while she was doing that, she'd also be able to use her resolve to keep her going until her new way of life became so internalized that it was automatic.

Different habits require different lengths of time to change. If, for example, you habitually drive on the right side of the road and then move to a country where people drive on the left, it would probably take you no more than a few days to change and internalize that habit. But if you're a smoker, it could take much longer to change that habit. My own experience has shown that to change our habitual eating and exercise patterns, we need to consciously repeat our new behaviors for thirty to forty days before they are transferred to the subconscious and become new habitual patterns. In fact, Sarah did internalize her new way of life. She lost more than sixty pounds in just three months, and she is now well on her way to achieving her goal weight of 125.

If you've watched any of the commercials for weight-loss programs that seem to be airing every ten minutes on television, you'll have noticed that virtually every one of them features a successful loser attesting to the fact that she (because it's almost always a woman) is *never going to go back* to what she was doing before. What those people are saying is that their new diet and exercise plan has become a permanent and automatic part of their lifestyle. And in many instances, they also describe some triggering event that got them started in the first place. It might have been the embarrassment of having to ask for a seat belt extender on a plane—and the vow never to be so embarrassed again. Or maybe it was a mother's realization that her ten-year-old daughter was in danger of becoming anorexic because she didn't want to grow up to look like her overweight mom—and the vow that the mother would start to model a healthier relationship with food.

In each of these instances, the triggering event was the discovery of a true core desire that unleashed the dieter's power of intention to change. But if you could question these people, they would undoubtedly also tell you that it took a while for the changes they made to become so ritualistic that they no longer required constant vigilance.

This means that for the first four to six weeks after you put your plan into action, you will have to apply your resolve and *consciously decide to stick with it every day.* After that time, it will become what I like to call a personal ritual, which is a kind of sacred act you perform for yourself not just because you think you should do it, but because it is internalized and has become part of your core being.

Resistance to Change

As I said at the beginning of this book, we humans are intrinsically resistant to change, and we are also fearful of the unknown. The anxiety we feel when we begin to change or venture into the unknown is actually our protective mechanism, and it can cause us—at least initially—to misinterpret or fail to recognize what is, in fact, a core desire.

To see how this works, imagine that a stranger is ringing your doorbell. The family dog becomes instantly alert and is ready to jump on whoever is about to come into your home. The stranger represents change, and the dog is your protective mechanism. Consciously, you may think that the stranger is there for a good purpose, but subconsciously, your instinct is to be afraid. The key, then, is to calm your dog down so that the person can safely come in. After a while, if the person is truly well-intentioned, the dog will get used to him and will no longer try to attack him. But if you were wrong in your initial assessment, the dog will know it and will continue to try to protect you. If that happens, your original plan of action may need adjusting. Being aware of how your protective dog works will enable you to venture into change smoothly and safely.

When you embark on any process of change, your brain will release neurotransmitters that create anxiety. The anxiety may be letting you know that what you're doing (allowing a stranger into your house) is wrong, but it may also be preventing you from letting in something (or someone) that is going to make your life better. Think of this in terms of accepting a new job. It may be the opportunity of a lifetime and the job of your dreams. You may be very excited about succeeding in the new job, but you are also, quite naturally, anxious about making the change. Continuing to visualize and affirm your goal (succeeding in the job of your dreams) will help you quiet your natural anxiety and move forward. In fact, just knowing that anxiety is a naturally occurring mental reaction to change will allow you to push through it and move forward until the unfamiliar becomes familiar and, therefore, no longer anxiety-producing. Remember this bit of wisdom: Change is the only constant in our lives.

Learning by Doing

We've already talked about how much of our life is driven by what's stored in our subconscious. If we aren't careful, those subconscious thoughts, beliefs, and associations can pop up at any moment like an action figure in a video game to hijack our conscious intentions and cut us off from following through on our plans.

Let's say, for example, you're on your way to lunch. You've planned to have a nice grilled chicken salad on a bed of greens with fresh lemon juice or dressing on the side. You're a block from the office when you pass the local hamburger joint, and the aroma of grilling burgers and French fries is more than you can resist. In an instant, your action plan is cast aside, and you succumb to the temptation.

Why does that happen? Probably because somewhere in your subconscious, you've stored the memory of the first time you had a burger and fries and how much you enjoyed that meal. It's not the aroma itself that got to you, because without the subconscious memory of enjoyment that's associated with that aroma, it wouldn't be meaningful, it wouldn't have the power to tempt you. You've *learned through experience* to associate the smell of a burger with something that's pleasurable. If you doubt that, consider the fact that some people don't like burgers, and the wafting aroma doesn't have the same power over them that it does over you.

In fact, almost everything we do without conscious thought has been learned—even brushing our teeth. You don't get up in the morning and have to consciously decide whether you're going to brush that day. You just do it. But as a little kid, you didn't automatically get out of bed and go into the bathroom to brush your teeth. Your mother first had to teach you how to do it, then she probably supervised you as you brushed, and when she was sure you'd learned how, she reminded you (you probably called it nagging) until brushing your teeth finally became part of your automatic routine.

On a physical level, walking through a door without bumping into the frame is something our bodies "remember" because we learned it through repetition when we first started to toddle around on our own. As a baby, you learned to stand up by trying and falling down over and over again. Now you don't consciously think about balancing each time you stand up; it's something your body does automatically. The same thing will be true of your new lifestyle. The more you practice it, the more firmly embedded in your subconscious it will become.

To keep on practicing your new eating and exercise patterns until they become as automatic as standing up and walking, you will need to call upon all the techniques we've been discussing. Use visualizations to remind yourself how great it will feel to reach your goal. Keep affirming to yourself that you can do it. Find a good trainer to coach and mentor you. Surround yourself with supportive people. Keep the workout appointments you make with yourself. Remember that you've signed an agreement with yourself to remain committed and do whatever it takes.

The Power of Consciousness

Up to this point, I've been emphasizing the power of the subconscious, but now I'd like to talk about the power of consciousness, which you'll be using initially to fuel your resolve. Because your creative ability rests in your mind, whatever you create—and that includes a new, healthier you—is a matter of will. The conscious mind makes decisions. It's what gives us free will, and it's what we can use to accept or reject the messages being triggered by the subconscious (like the smell of that hamburger) while we're working toward establishing new automatic behaviors.

When it comes to changing your eating and exercise habits, free will and will-power go hand in hand. It's your free will that allows you to exercise the willpower to reject the allure of the burger or overcome the temptation to skip your workout on any given day. I know what you're thinking: *I've tried to use willpower before and it's worked for a while, but in the end I just gave in and went back to my old bad habits.*

Well, that was before you knew what you know now.

- You've already reframed your fitness goal in terms of achieving a true core desire, which is bigger and more powerful than just wanting to lose weight and get fit.
- You've made an appropriate plan.
- You have the tools you need to fuel the power of your intention.
- You're working on overwriting those old negative tapes that have been preventing your body from becoming what you want it to be.

And now you know that you're not going to have to depend on your willpower forever, because in just thirty to forty days, your new behavioral patterns will be internalized and will become your personal ritual.

Until your new lifestyle becomes habitual, there will be many of those tempting burger moments, and one of the most powerful tools you have to resist them is to become aware of how you feel when you think about giving in to temptation.

There are many ways to analyze and interpret our thoughts, but there are only two ways we can *feel*—good or bad. When we feel good, we are excited. When we feel bad, we are anxious or fearful. Think of your feelings as traffic lights, letting you know whether to proceed or to stop until the danger passes. When you come to a curb and see a green light, you know it's safe to cross the street. If the light is red, you know you need to stop and wait to avoid being run over.

Imagine that you've scheduled a session at the gym after work, but then you receive a call from a friend inviting you to join her for a drink. Because your new habits have not yet become automatic, you accept the invitation and decide to skip your workout. By doing that, you're letting yourself down, and you're probably feeling some anxiety. But because you really want to go out and have a good time, you may be pushing down and ignoring that feeling. So the next time you're tempted to skip a workout and have a drink, or go directly home and relax in front of the TV because you're tired, stop and let yourself really feel the feeling that comes up in conjunction with that decision.

Because the feeling always follows directly upon the thought, being mindful of what you are feeling in the moment can prevent you from taking the action—going out for that drink or going home to watch television—that will only make you feel worse in the long run. The more conscious you become of your feelings, the more easily you'll be able to identify them, and the less likely you'll be to push them down and engage in the activity that you know subconsciously, on the level of feeling, you shouldn't be doing in the first place.

The More You Practice, the Easier It Gets

Juliene Berk, author of *The Down Comforter*, writes, "Habits . . . the only reason they persist is that they are offering some satisfaction. . . . You allow them to persist by not seeking any other, better form of satisfying the same needs. Every habit, good or bad, is acquired and learned in the same way—by finding that it is a means of satisfaction."

"Practice makes perfect" isn't just an old adage. Many psychologists believe that people will learn a new habit only if it benefits them, and the longer you practice your new behaviors, the more you will begin to see the benefits. Your success will fuel future successes, and with each passing day, sticking with your program is going to get easier.

Why? First, because the better you get at it, the less difficult it will be. That's one of the reasons I've said that your original plan of action may have to be changed or amended. If you think about Sarah for a minute, you'll realize that the exercise routine we worked out when she weighed more than two hundred pounds wasn't going to be as effective as she lost weight, gained muscle, and became capable of doing much more than she could initially.

Beyond that, as you begin to see the fruits of your labor, you'll have much greater belief in your ability to succeed. Not only will that belief increase your chances of succeeding, but it also will inspire you to do better and better.

Success becomes a self-fulfilling prophecy and actually shifts your subconscious expectations for yourself. The mental and physical aspects of your life work in tandem to create the person you become.

What If You Slip Up?

Actually, that shouldn't be phrased as a question, because you will no doubt slip up from time to time, especially during the initial four to six weeks while your new behaviors are becoming internalized. After all, you're human, not a robot. But slipping up doesn't mean giving up. Now you know you can use the meditations, affirmations, and visualizations that have been fueling the power of your intention to relieve the unavoidable stress that can work to undermine your best intentions, to reaffirm your resolve, and to refocus on how you will feel when you've achieved your true core desire. In other words, when the going gets tough, you need to reach deep within yourself and keep your eyes on the prize.

Let's Go!

Now, armed with your true core desire, the power of your intention, your action plan, and your resolve to make it happen, it's time to get started. In the following chapter, I'll provide you with an easy-to-follow, simple-to-implement eating plan that balances lean protein with complex carbohydrates and good, heart-healthy fats. You'll be eating every three hours, so you'll never be hungry, which will make it easier for you to resist temptation. And by following this plan as you also begin to exercise, you'll be simultaneously losing fat and building muscle. As you're about to learn, increasing your muscle mass—not just losing excess body fat—is the key to becoming lean, fit, and healthy.

HOW TO EAT WELL AND EXERCISE RIGHT WITHOUT GIVING UP YOUR LIFE

Five

The 40/40/20 × 5 Fat-Loss Plan

As your perception is, so will your action be. The thing to change is not your action but your outlook. What must I do to change it? Merely understand that your present way of looking is defective.
—Anthony De Mello, *Awareness*

When Amanda walked into my office, she appeared to be in her mid-forties. At about five foot two and one hundred pounds, she was also a little too skinny. But the most striking thing about her was how nervous and "hyper" she seemed. She was speaking so quickly that I could hardly understand her, and her hands were visibly shaking.

I generally start each session with a new client by doing a relaxation exercise, but Amanda was anxious to get right to the fitness assessment. When I took her blood pressure, we were both astonished to discover that it was extremely high, and her heart was beating so quickly that I wanted to send her to see a doctor that very minute. Amanda, however, insisted that we continue with the consultation. She'd been working with a trainer for the past three years, and what she really wanted was for "Mr. Universe" to tell her how great she was doing.

I explained that, ethically, because of her elevated blood pressure and rapid heart beat, I couldn't put her through a strength or aerobics test and suggested that we just talk about her nutritional habits. Her percentage of body fat was too low to be considered healthy, and when I asked how many meals she was eating each day, she said two, lunch and a protein bar. I couldn't stop myself from asking why she was undereating. Her response was that, in her opinion, she was *overeating*. Although Amanda wasn't, strictly speaking, anorexic, she was certainly well on her way to becoming so.

She shared with me that she regularly suffered from headaches and that, from time to time, she felt short of breath. As she was getting up to leave, she asked me about a weight-loss product she was taking. Although I'd asked her at the beginning of our session if she was taking any medications or supplements, this one had apparently slipped her mind. The product contained ephedra (which has only recently been taken off the market), and I said, "Amanda, I'm not a doctor, but in my opinion this product is undoubtedly one of the causes—if not the primary cause—of your high blood pressure and elevated heart rate. My advice to you is to stop taking it immediately and to see your doctor as soon as possible."

With that, she threw the bottle in the trash and, with tears in her eyes, hugged me so hard I thought she would break. When she walked out of my office, her one desire was to save her life.

For some people, looking good is worth the price of poor health. My point in telling you this story is to let you know that you can be fit, happy, and healthy without killing yourself. That is true whether you're overweight and out of shape or, like Amanda, underweight and equally unhealthy.

You'll be hearing more about Amanda in the following chapter, but for now you should know that after she was off her weight-loss product for a few weeks, her blood pressure and heart rate returned to normal. With her fitness goal shifted to focus on good health and by following my nutritional plan, she gained fifteen pounds, and both her weight and body fat are now ideal for her height, age, and bone structure. Most important, she's happy, and she feels great.

Think About How Far You've Come

It took a real health scare to change Amanda's approach to fitness and health, but it needn't be that way. Before you begin to implement the nutrition and exercise plans I'm about to provide, I want you to take some time to consider how much you've already changed your outlook. By rethinking your goals in terms of a core desire, you've changed your entire approach to weight loss and fitness. You've rethought the way you spend your time in order to create more balance in your life. By learning how to meditate, visualize your achievement, and affirm your ability to succeed, you've acquired some powerful tools to ensure that you'll do whatever it takes to honor your commitment. And you now understand that because your body is the servant of your mind, using these mental exercises will change the way your body behaves. The power of your mind is also the reason you need to change the way you've probably thought about weight-loss programs in the past.

Become Conscious of What You're Thinking

Since *Mind Over Body* is all about using your mind to change your body, I suggest that before you go any further, you check in with your subconscious to see whether you still harbor any of the following beliefs. To make sure that you're really focused and in touch with your thoughts, do the deep-breathing exercise on page 19. Now, consider which of the following statements reflect your own beliefs.

- I feel tired; I need food.
- I know everything about exercising and eating healthily; I'll start next week.
- I love food too much; I'll never be able to stick with this diet.
- I have tried before and failed every time; I am not strong enough mentally.
- I will never be able to concentrate on my work if I have to starve every day.
- My husband (or my wife, or my partner) cooks so well, I can't resist.
- We always go out to eat; it's impossible to diet when you're eating in restaurants.
- Weekends are times to eat.
- I'll start my diet Monday.
- I am stressed, and stress makes me eat more.
- If I eat more today, I'll work out more tomorrow.
- I love my beers too much after dinner, when I'm sitting in front of the TV.
- No way I will give up ice cream after dinner.
- I travel for my job, and I have to stay in hotels and eat what's available.
- I am overweight, but I am happy; why would I change who I am?

Once you become aware of these thoughts and understand how they are causing you to behave, you can use the affirmations and meditation techniques you've already learned to turn your mind around so that your body will follow.

How to Think About This Plan

The best piece of advice I can give you is this: Don't think of this as a diet. A diet is something people go "on" to lose weight and then "off" until they gain the weight back, at which point they go "on" the diet again. You've probably done that yourself at least a few times in the past. I, too, have been on diets. When I was a professional bodybuilder, I did some crazy and sometimes unsafe things to my body in order to compete. One of the dumbest things I ever did was, at the age of twenty-one, to stop drinking water for seventy-two hours before a competition so that I would look super-lean or, as we say in the bodybuilding world, "ripped." Why would I do such a thing? Because one of my teammates suggested it. I would have wound up in the hospital instead of onstage if my own instincts—not to mention the fact that I appeared to be shrinking by the minute and was feeling horrible—hadn't told me to drink. Within hours I was back to normal. I didn't win the competition (I did come in second), but I learned a good lesson.

I haven't done anything that crazy since, and I haven't "dieted" since my last competition in 1991. Since then, I've been following a balanced, healthy nutritional plan very similar to the one I'll give you. It's a way to eat for the rest of your life.

In addition to the on-again, off-again nature of diets, they can also be physically and emotionally harmful. Many diets are so restrictive that they cause you to lose muscle mass and slow down your metabolism, actually encouraging your body to store fat instead of burning it. They can also create vitamin and mineral deficiencies that leave you fatigued and craving the very starchy, sugary foods you should be avoiding.

Think of this program as a fat-loss plan, not a weight-loss plan. Excess weight or weight gain is not actually the problem; it's a symptom of the underlying problem, which is the accumulation of unhealthy body fat. And the cause of excess body fat is a lack of muscle. Therefore, this plan concentrates on building muscle and losing fat—forever.

Very often people who come to consult with me say that they're thirty pounds overweight. I look at them and tell them they're wrong. In actuality, they're probably carrying forty pounds of excess fat and lacking thirty pounds of muscle. When I suggest this, most people are surprised—they never thought of the various kinds of tissue that contribute to their total body weight.

As many of us know, a pound of fat has more than twice the volume of a pound of muscle. But think about what this actually means: By changing the ratio of muscle to fat in your body, you'll actually weigh more but look thinner. If, for example, you weigh 135 pounds but have only 24 pounds of body fat, you'll easily fit into clothing that someone who is the same weight but has 40 pounds of body fat couldn't possibly wear.

In addition to how you look, your ratio of muscle to fat can have a profound impact on your overall health and fitness. In fact, many of the health issues associated with excess body fat—chronic fatigue syndrome, lower back pain, high blood pressure, and high cholesterol, to name just a few—actually result from a loss of muscle. The higher your percentage of body fat, the lower your percentage of muscle, and vice versa.

You Need Some Fat to Stay Alive

People often ask me what my percentage of body fat was when I became Mr. Universe. The answer is 3 percent, but that was probably for no more than a couple of days, after which it went back to somewhere between 5 and 7 percent. Assuming you're not a professional bodybuilder, that percentage would be unrealistic for you.

We all need some fat just to maintain cellular structure, regulate body temperature, cushion and insulate our organs, and store the energy we need to stay alive. The following table indicates the average range of body fat for men and women in various categories.

Category	Women	Men
Vital fat (necessary to maintain life)	10 to 12 percent	3 to 5 percent
Athlete	13 to 19 percent	6 to 13 percent
Fit	20 to 24 percent	14 to 17 percent
Average	25 to 31 percent	18 to 25 percent
Obese	32 percent or more	26 percent or more

Note that women naturally have a higher percentage of body fat than men—6 to 7 percent more. By nature, a woman's body is made to protect a potential fetus. As a result, women have more enzymes than men for storing fat and fewer enzymes for burning fat. Furthermore, the estrogen in a woman's system activates fat-storing enzymes and causes them to multiply. Another difference between men and women is that most women store fat below the waist—in their buttocks, hips, and thighs—whereas most men store it primarily in their abdomen, lower back, and chest. Many studies have shown that the woman's pattern of fat storage is generally healthier than the man's, and that excess abdominal fat indicates an increased risk for developing heart disease.

IF YOU WANT TO LEARN YOUR PERCENTAGE OF BODY FAT . . .

Although determining your percentage of body fat isn't necessary for following this plan, it can be both interesting and useful to do so before you begin.

You can do this by using calipers designed for the purpose. If you wish, you can buy the calipers (the Acumeasure brand costs about $15), follow the instructions, and take the measurements yourself. Or—my preference—you can go to a gym and have the measurements done professionally. The American College of Sports Medicine has stated that skinfold measurements, when performed by a trained tester, are very accurate measures of body fat.

Measuring your body fat before you start the plan and then at intervals as you progress can be very validating and motivating, as you'll see the percentage decline.

My reason for telling you all this about body fat is to help you understand why it's so important not only to cut calories but also to eat a proper balance of nutrients that will help you build muscle while you lose weight. The eating plan in this chapter is designed specifically to help you do just that.

Determine Your *"Ideal"* Weight

Before you start this fat-loss journey, you'll need to know where you want to end up. Please notice that I've put the word *ideal* in quotation marks. That's because I don't want you to think of it as the weight you *must* aim to reach. The following charts were created by the Metropolitan Life Insurance Company based on statistics associated with the lowest risk of mortality. However, each person is unique; no two have exactly the same bone structure or body composition, and some have particular health issues or other concerns that need to be considered. Therefore, you must consider what weight will make you feel comfortable and fit. You also need to be realistic. If you haven't weighed at the low end of the range for your height since you hit puberty, that target is probably not realistic. Don't set yourself up for failure by pursuing a goal that your body isn't capable of achieving.

HEIGHT AND WEIGHT TABLE FOR WOMEN			
Height	Small Frame	Medium Frame	Large Frame
4' 10"	102–111	109–121	118–131
4' 11"	103–113	111–123	120–134
5' 0"	104–115	113–126	122–137
5' 1"	106–118	115–129	125–140
5' 2"	108–121	118–132	128–143
5' 3"	111–124	121–135	131–147
5' 4"	114–127	124–138	134–151
5' 5"	117–130	127–141	137–155
5' 6"	120–133	130–144	140–159
5' 7"	123–136	133–147	143–163
5' 8"	126–139	136–150	146–167
5' 9"	129–142	139–153	149–170
5' 10"	132–145	142–156	152–173
5' 11"	135–148	145–159	155–176
6' 0"	138–151	148–162	158–179

Weights at ages 25–59 based on lowest mortality. Weight in pounds according to frame (in indoor clothing weighing 3 pounds; shoes with 1-inch heels).

Reprinted with the permission of MetLife. This information is not intended to be a substitute for professional medical advice and should not be regarded as an endorsement or approval of any product or service.

HEIGHT AND WEIGHT TABLE FOR MEN

Height	Small Frame	Medium Frame	Large Frame
5′ 2″	128–134	131–141	138–150
5′ 3″	130–136	133–143	140–153
5′ 4″	132–138	135–145	142–156
5′ 5″	134–140	137–148	144–160
5′ 6″	136–142	139–151	146–164
5′ 7″	138–145	142–154	149–168
5′ 8″	140–148	145–157	152–172
5′ 9″	142–151	148–160	155–176
5′ 10″	144–154	151–163	158–180
5′ 11″	146–157	154–166	161–184
6′ 0″	149–160	157–170	164–188
6′ 1″	152–164	160–174	168–192
6′ 2″	155–168	164–178	172–197
6′ 3″	158–172	167–182	176–202
6′ 4″	162–176	171–187	181–207

Weights at ages 25–59 based on lowest mortality. Weight in pounds according to frame (in indoor clothing weighing 3 lbs.; shoes with 1″ heels).

Reprinted with the permission of MetLife. This information is not intended to be a substitute for professional medical advice and should not be regarded as an endorsement or approval of any product or service.

The size of your frame is based on the circumference of your wrist with relation to your height. Measure your wrist with a tape measure and use the following chart to determine the size of your frame.

FRAME SIZE: WOMEN

Frame	Height		
	Under 5'2"	5'2" to 5'5"	Over 5'5"
Small	Wrist < 5.5"	Wrist < 6"	Wrist < 6.25"
Medium	Wrist 5.5"–5.75"	Wrist 6"–6.25"	Wrist 6.25"–6.5"
Large	Wrist >5.75"	Wrist > 6.25"	Wrist 6.5"

FRAME SIZE: MEN

Frame	Height over 5'5"
Small	Wrist 5.5"–6.5"
Medium	Wrist 6.5"–7.5"
Large	Wrist > 7.5"

Now that you have a target to shoot for, I'll show you how to get there.

Determine How Many Calories You Need to Reach Your Ideal Weight

With your current weight and target weight in mind, you need to do a bit of figuring before you get started. First you need to determine your basal metabolic rate (BMR), which is the amount of energy (or number of calories) you require to fuel your most basic bodily functions—breathing, pumping blood through your veins, thinking, sweating, talking, and so on. To do that, women need to multiply their weight by 10, and men need to multiply it by 11. For example, if you are a woman and your weight is 150 pounds, 150 × 10 = 1500. Your BMR is 1500. That means you burn approximately 1500 calories at rest. If you are a man and your weight is 180 pounds, 180 × 11 = 1980. Your BMR is 1980.

Add the Activity Factor

Your BMR is the number of calories you need just to stay alive, but I'm assuming that you want to do more than that. You get to add calories based on your level of activity.

Sedentary (little or no exercise, desk job): Multiply your BMR by 1.2.

Light activity (light exercise/activity, 20 minutes 1 to 3 days a week): Multiply your BMR by 1.3.

Moderate activity (moderate exercise/activity, 30 to 60 minutes 3 to 5 days a week): Multiply your BMR by 1.4.

Heavy activity (heavy exercise/activity, 60 to 90 minutes 6 to 7 days a week): Multiply your BMR by 1.5.

If you are a woman with a BMR of 1500 and are moderately active (using the exercise program in the following chapter, for example), you need to multiply 1500 by 1.4 to determine the total number of calories required to maintain your weight:

$1500 \times 1.4 = 2100$. I call this your total calorie requirement (TCR). If you are a man with a BMR of 1980 and are moderately active, you need to multiply 1980 by 1.4 to determine your TCR: $1980 \times 1.4 = 2772$.

Now you know the number of calories it takes to maintain your current weight. *To lose weight, you'll need to reduce that number by 500 calories.* So for the examples above, the woman should eat 1600 calories per day and the man 2272.

One pound of body fat equals 3500 calories. So if you reduce your calorie intake by 500 calories a day, even if you don't increase your activity level, you'll be losing one pound of body fat per week.

As you increase muscle tone and lose fat, your metabolism will increase, which means that you will begin to burn more calories and therefore lose weight even more quickly.

One pound of body fat burns 3 calories a day.

One pound of muscle burns 50 calories a day.

A word of warning: Don't think that if you restrict your calories even more, you'll lose weight faster. If you consume fewer than 1200 calories per day, your body will be fooled into thinking it's starving and will automatically begin to metabolize calories more slowly to conserve energy.

Consider Your Age

As you age, you may become less active. You may sit more, exercise less vigorously, and perform less physical labor. Your metabolism may also slow down and become less efficient. With each decade, starting at age thirty, muscle mass declines, which means that you burn fewer calories. Exercise and physical activity such as strength training can help to increase muscle mass and raise your metabolism.

The 40/40/20 × 5 Fat-Loss Plan

Now that you know how many calories you should be consuming to arrive at your goal weight, it's time to determine how those calories should be distributed and what foods you should be eating to build the most muscle and burn the most fat. On the 40/40/20 × 5 Fat-Loss Plan, you won't have to eat any specific foods at any specific meal. You'll always have plenty to choose from, which means that you won't be bored, and you'll be able to eat out and enjoy your meal without worrying about going off the plan.

It's really as simple as 1, 2, 3.

1. *For every meal, think 40/40/20.* Forty percent of your diet should consist of carbohydrates that are low to moderate on the Glycemic Index (those that are absorbed more slowly and therefore do not spike blood sugar levels), 40 percent of proteins of high biological value (those that are most easily digested, are quickly absorbed by the cells, and most closely match the types of protein found in the body), and 20 percent of heart-healthy fats. You can also eat as many foods as you want from the "free" list on page 107.

2. *Stick to the correct portion sizes.* A "portion" for most of us is a lot less food than we're accustomed to being served, particularly in a restaurant. To determine the correct portion size for you, see pages 111–112.

3. *Eat five small meals a day at three-hour intervals.* By doing this, you'll ensure that you're never "starving" and your blood sugar will remain level. As a result, you won't be tempted to overeat or to grab the first fatty, sugary snack that crosses your path.

If you follow these three simple rules, you can expect to lose between one and three pounds of fat per week, depending on your activity level, and you won't have to work out like a maniac to do it. You'll have a steady source of energy from morning to night, your brain will be sharp, and your body will be strong.

YOUR 40/40/20 × 5
MIND-OVER-BODY DAY

6:00 a.m.: Shower

6:15 a.m.: Morning meditation and affirmations

7:00 a.m.: Workout session; **1 small piece of fruit before exercising** (Exercising in the morning helps boost your metabolism.)

7:30 a.m.: **Meal 1:** Breakfast

8:00 a.m.: Get ready to go to office

10:30 a.m.: **Meal 2:** Midmorning snack

12:30 or 1:00 p.m.: **Meal 3:** Lunch

1:30 p.m.: Back to office

4:30 p.m.: **Meal 4:** Midafternoon snack

5:00 p.m.: Free time

7:30 p.m.: **Meal 5:** Dinner

9:00 p.m.: Unwind; quality time with family or by yourself

10:00 p.m.: Bedtime; visualization and affirmations for 10 minutes

10:15 p.m.: Sweet dreams!

Why Breakfast Is Important

If you skip breakfast, you'll be putting yourself in starvation mode before the day has even begun. Not only do people who skip breakfast burn fewer calories than those who eat a balanced morning meal, but they also tend to eat more starchy, sugary, nutrient-poor calories at the next meal because they're so hungry and need a quick energy boost. I remember the days when I went to school without breakfast. Not only was I worn-out both mentally and physically by 10 a.m., but I was so hungry by lunchtime that I could have devoured an elephant.

The Best 40/40/20 Foods to Choose

It is important to get the most out of what you eat. My belief is that the closer foods are to their natural state, the better they are for you. With that in mind, I generally recommend getting the bulk of your calories from foods such as brown rice, plain oatmeal, sweet potatoes, fish, chicken breasts, turkey, fresh fruits, and steamed fresh vegetables. Eating these types of foods will provide you with sustained energy throughout the day.

Good Carbs: 40 Percent of Calories

I'm sure you've heard about "simple" and "complex" carbohydrates, but you may not know exactly what those terms mean or why they're significant.

All carbohydrates are sugars, starches, and fibers made up of chains of carbon and water. The chains vary in length, and those comprising the shortest chains—mainly sugars and refined starches—are called simple. Longer-chain carbohydrates—mainly unrefined starches and fiber—are complex.

When any type of carbohydrate is digested, it is turned into glucose in your bloodstream (which causes your blood sugar level to rise). When your body senses glucose in the bloodstream, it releases insulin, which causes the excess glucose to be absorbed from the bloodstream and either used for energy or stored as fat (causing your blood sugar level to fall).

Short-chain, simple carbohydrates are digested quickly, causing your blood glucose and insulin levels to rise and fall very rapidly. This rapid fluctuation leaves you feeling tired, headachy, and irritable and leads you to crave more simple carbs to raise your blood sugar again and give you another quick energy boost. Long-chain, complex carbohydrates, which take longer to digest, release glucose more slowly and steadily, keeping your blood sugar level steady, which means that your mood and your energy will also remain steady throughout the day.

Other than the "free" vegetables listed on page 107, the carbs I recommend are those that are low to moderate on the Glycemic Index (GI). These are the carbs you digest slowly, so that they don't cause fluctuations in blood sugar levels. I suggest that you choose the majority of your carbs from those that are low on the GI.

Fruits	GI
Apples	low
Apricots	medium
Bananas (yellow, ripe)	medium
Blueberries	low
Cantaloupe	medium
Cherries	low
Grapefruit	low
Mangoes	low
Oranges	low
Papaya	medium
Peaches	low
Pears	low
Pineapple	low
Plums	low
Prunes	medium
Raisins	medium
Strawberries	low

Vegetables	GI
Beans (also contain more than 20% protein and less than 20% fat)	low
Beets	medium
Carrots, raw or cooked	low
Lentils (also contain more than 20% protein and less than 20% fat)	low
Soybeans (also contain more than 20% protein and less than 20% fat)	low

Starches and Grains	GI
Brown rice	low
Corn tortillas	low
Oatmeal	medium
Oat bran	low
Pasta (preferably whole wheat)	low
Whole barley	low
Whole grain breads	medium
Yam or sweet potato	low

WHAT DOES THE GLYCEMIC INDEX REALLY MEAN?

The Glycemic Index (GI) is a system for ranking foods—specifically carbohydrates—according to how they affect your blood sugar level. Those that are "low" on the GI create a slow, steady rise that's easy on the body. The higher on the GI the food is rated, the more quickly it raises blood sugar. The faster blood sugar goes up, however, the faster it falls, and your energy level falls with it. That leads to cravings for more of the fast-working—mainly starchy, sugary—carbs that will give you the quick energy you need. You'll notice that there are no foods that are high on the GI in the list on pages 102–103. The aim of the 40/40/20 × 5 Fat-Loss Plan is to keep your blood sugar—and energy—level steady throughout the day.

Proteins of High Biological Value: 40 Percent of Calories

Animal sources such as meat, poultry, fish, and egg whites provide proteins of high biological value (proteins that are most easily digested and absorbed into the cells and that are closest to those found in the human body) and should comprise the bulk of your protein calories.

Food	Biological Value
Beans	45
Beef (lean)	80
Chicken breast (skinless)	84
Egg whites	104
Fish (tuna, flounder, halibut, cod, salmon)	75
Milk protein	72
Nuts	40
Quinoa	71
Soy protein	74
Whey protein	130

WHAT IS QUINOA?

Sometimes called the "perfect food," quinoa is a unique whole grain grown in South America that is a complete protein, containing all the essential amino acids that the body cannot manufacture and must obtain from food sources. Originally used by the Incas, it can be substituted for rice in almost any recipe.

ADDITIONAL GOOD PROTEIN SOURCES

Crab	Lobster (steamed)
Duck	Low-fat cottage cheese
Lean ground turkey	Shrimp (steamed)
Lean ham	Soy milk
Lean pork	Venison

Good Fats: 20 Percent of Calories

Good fats are the monounsaturated and polyunsaturated fats that can actually help to lower cholesterol levels.

Monounsaturated Fats

Avocados	Olives
Canola oil	Nuts
Olive oil	Peanut oil

Polyunsaturated Fats

Corn oil	Soybean oil
Omega-3 fatty acids	Sunflower oil
Safflower oil	

WHAT ARE OMEGA-3 FATTY ACIDS?

These are essential fatty acids, meaning that we can't manufacture them and must obtain them from food sources. Found mainly in fatty fish such as salmon, omega-3 fatty acids have been shown to benefit healthy people as well as those who are at risk for (or already have) cardiovascular disease. According to Dr. Michael Colgan, author of *Optimum Sports Nutrition*, they can also help regulate insulin metabolism.

Free Foods

You may eat as much of these foods as you like throughout the day.

All extracts

All dry seasonings and fresh herbs

All vegetables *except* corn, parsnips, squash, carrots, and beets

Crystal Light

Decaffeinated coffee or tea

Flavored waters, such as fruit and/or vitamin waters

   (Avoid those that contain artificial sweeteners.)

Lemon and lime juice

Regular coffee or tea (consult with your physician for the amount you are allowed)

Sauces and condiments, such as barbecue sauce, teriyaki sauce, soy sauce

   (low sodium), A.1. sauce, mustard, relish, and salsa

Vinegars

WATER, THE FORGOTTEN NUTRIENT

Water is actually the most important nutrient you can feed your body. It aids digestion, carries nutrients and oxygen throughout the body, and transports waste material for elimination. In addition, it lubricates your joints, protects your organs, and helps maintain a normal body temperature. It's used by every cell, and many of your most important biochemical reactions and metabolic processes do not occur efficiently unless you are well hydrated.

Poor hydration can make you tired, prevent your brain from functioning at its peak, and slow your metabolism. Sometimes when you think you're hungry, you may really just be thirsty. Many Americans are chronically dehydrated.

On average, your body loses 8 to 12 cups of water a day, and that amount increases when the weather is hot, when you exercise, when you increase your fiber intake, and when you drink caffeinated beverages or alcohol.

Women generally need to replace 8 to 10 cups of water a day, and men need to replace 12 cups. In addition to water, you get fluids from the following sources.

- Decaffeinated coffee or tea
- Fresh fruits and vegetables
- Fruit juice
- Most meats
- Nonalcoholic beer
- Skim milk
- Soup

Keep bottles of water on your desk and in your car. Keep a pitcher of water in the refrigerator. Drink a glass of water before each meal and snack. Drink a cup of water after each cup of coffee or other caffeinated beverage.

Foods to *Avoid* on the 40/40/20 Plan

Carbohydrates

All cereals (except oat bran and oatmeal)

Bagels (except whole wheat)

Foods with added sugar

Fruit bars (energy bars that are loaded with sugar)

Fruit juice

Soda (except 1 diet soda a day)

IS IT OKAY TO DRINK DIET SODA?

According to a study conducted at the University of Texas Health Science Center at San Antonio, there appears to be an association between drinking diet soda and weight gain. The study followed more than six hundred normal-weight people and discovered that after eight years those who drank one diet soda a day were 65 percent more likely to have become overweight than those who drank regular soda.

The study didn't actually indicate that drinking diet soda *caused* weight gain, but the association was significant. There is some speculation that artificial sweeteners may cause us to crave the real thing. Another possibility might be that those who drink diet soda feel that they can compensate for the calories saved by eating more high-calorie foods.

> I believe it's okay to drink one diet soda a day if you crave the sweet taste, so long as you avoid those that contain caffeine and/or saccharine. You're better off sticking with plain or flavored water, however.

Proteins

Fatty meats (all pork, lamb, and beef *except* cuts from the loin)

Fatty dairy foods (such as whole milk, cheese, and egg yolks)

Most luncheon meats (contain high amounts of sodium that cause you to retain water)

Fats

Saturated fats, found primarily in foods from animal sources, including dairy products (cheese, whole milk, and butter) and meat (chicken, beef, and pork)

BUTTER OR MARGARINE—WHICH ONE IS BETTER?

Butter is a saturated fat. A stick of butter contains as much fat and cholesterol—and double the amount of saturated fat—as *three* quarter-pound burgers with cheese!

Margarine generally has much less saturated fat than butter, but that can be in the form of trans fat, which is created when liquid vegetable oils are hydrogenated to make them more solid.

Trans fat raises "bad" LDL cholesterol and lowers "good" HDL cholesterol. The American Heart Association recommends using only margarines that contain less than 2 percent saturated fat.

How to Determine the Proper Portion Size

You now know *what* foods you should be choosing, but you're probably wondering *how much* of each one you should be eating at each meal.

To figure that out, begin with the number of calories you've determined you should be consuming each day to lose weight. Divide that number by 5—the number of meals you'll be eating. Now you know how many calories you can consume at each meal.

Using our previous examples (see pages 97–98):

Woman = 1600 ÷ 5 = 320 calories per meal

Man = 2272 ÷ 5 = 454 calories per meal

Remember that 40 percent of your calories at each meal will be coming from carbohydrates, 40 percent from protein, and 20 percent from fat. The easiest way to figure these percentages is to divide the total number of calories per meal by 10, then multiply by 4 to get your carbohydrate and protein calories and by 2 to get your fat calories. So, for the woman who's eating 320 calories per meal, that would be 128 calories each of carbohydrate and protein per meal and 64 calories of fat.

But that still doesn't tell you what you need to know about portion size, right? One way to determine the quantity of each nutrient (carbs, protein, and fat) to put on your plate at each meal is to weigh your food.

1 gram carbohydrate = 4 calories

1 gram protein = 4 calories

1 gram fat = 9 calories

You can certainly do that if you want to, but you don't have to. Luckily, nature has provided a very easy way for you to determine your correct portion size without having to weigh or measure anything.

- A portion of carbohydrate is the size of your fist.
- A portion of protein is the size of your palm.
- A portion of fat is the length of your thumb from the first joint to the tip.

Why does this work? Because the bigger you are, the bigger your palm and fist are. The size of your body is telling you the size of the portion you should be eating.

How to Avoid Portion Distortion

Unfortunately, most Americans are so used to "super-sizing" everything that they no longer have any idea what a proper portion should look like. Portion sizes in fast-food restaurants are now three to five times larger than they were in the 1950s. This means that, at least initially, you may be worried that with my plan you're not going to be getting enough food to fill you up. In fact, because you'll be eating every three hours, you really don't have to be concerned about going hungry. But if you want to be on the safe side, you can fill half your plate with "free" vegetables. No one ever got fat from eating their vegetables!

If you're worried about overeating, determine the correct portion size before you cook your food, and don't prepare any extra. If it isn't there in front of you, you won't be tempted to eat it.

You can also fool the eye—and your mind—by using smaller plates. If your plate is full, your portions will appear more generous.

Why Eat Five Times a Day?

The most important reason to eat more frequent smaller meals is that you'll always be eating *before* you're ravenously hungry, which will make it much easier for you to control the amount you consume at each meal. You'll also be ensuring that your blood sugar level remains stable, which means that you won't be tempted to rev yourself up with sugary, starchy high-GI carbs.

But there are other important health reasons to eat small meals as well. A British study conducted at Cambridge University showed that people who ate several small meals instead of one or two large ones reduced their cholesterol by approximately 5 percent, even when they ate more total calories and more calories from fat than when they were eating larger meals. "Total cholesterol and low-density lipoprotein ['bad' LDL cholesterol] decreased in a continuous relation with increasing daily frequency of eating," states the report published in the *British Medical Journal.* "This finding was particularly striking in view of the increased [caloric] intake, including fat intake, in people who reported eating more frequently."

Of course, as Dr. Joseph Mercola, author of *Dr. Mercola's Total Health Program,* said when commenting on the research, "the extra food that is eaten should still be high quality food that does not disrupt your immune system and impair your insulin balance."

Another good reason to eat small meals is that when you take in calories from food, your body either uses them for energy or stores them as fat. If you eat too many calories at a single meal and don't expend them as energy, guess what happens? Those "extra" calories get stored as fat. So if you're concerned about weight loss, it makes sense not to eat more calories than you expend in any given period of time.

Realistically, you probably won't be eating *exactly* the same number of calories at every meal, but it's best to try to keep your meals as equal as possible. Most of you may be used to thinking of your midmorning and midafternoon meals as snacks. These may be as simple as a protein shake or bar or a small meal such as cottage cheese and nuts, but I call them meals because they should provide approximately the same number of calories as the other three meals, and they should contain protein and carbohydrates as well as a small amount of good fat. Think of your "snacks" as convenient, energizing meal replacements.

There are many brands of protein bars available, so try a few different ones until you find those you like best. Just read the labels carefully to be sure they don't contain excessive amounts of sugar and/or fat. You should be looking for bars that contain no more than 7 grams of sugar and 8 grams of fat.

Mindful Hunger

If you're a parent, you undoubtedly know that a baby cries when he or she is hungry. As an adult, you probably don't actually shed tears when you're hungry, but your body still cries out to be fed. You wouldn't ignore your baby's cry for food, and you shouldn't ignore your own either.

This plan asks you to eat five times a day, or approximately every three hours, because the surest way to overeat is to wait until you're absolutely famished. If you wait until you're "starving," you'll be gulping your food down, and you can easily eat up to 5000 calories before your brain has a chance to let your stomach know it's full. Use your mind to help your body by being aware of how hungry you are, and eat when you're at a 2 or 3 on the following scale.

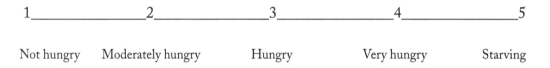

1	2	3	4	5
Not hungry	Moderately hungry	Hungry	Very hungry	Starving

Don't eat when you're not hungry, and don't wait to eat until you're very hungry or starving.

How Hungry Are You?

Very often people on restrictive diets feel hungry all the time because they've disconnected the mechanism by which the brain signals the body that it's full. As a result, they may be eating because they're stressed or upset, not because they're hungry. Here are a few tips for getting back in touch with your hunger signals.

- It takes twenty minutes from the time you start eating for the brain to signal the stomach that it's full. So if you eat too quickly, you'll overstuff yourself before that signal has time to arrive. Eat slowly and be mindful of what your brain is telling your body.
- If you think you're hungry, drink a glass of water and wait approximately fifteen minutes to see if you still feel hunger. If you drink a full glass of water before you begin each meal, you won't be confusing hunger with thirst.

- If you think you're hungry, try engaging in an activity you enjoy. You may discover that you were thinking about food only because you were bored, stressed, fatigued, or frustrated with what you were doing.
- If you're craving something sweet, wait fifteen minutes. Involve yourself in an activity or engage in conversation, and more often than not your craving will pass. If you still crave a sweet after fifteen minutes, try eating a healthier alternative, such as sugar-free frozen yogurt. Or eat just a small amount of the food you crave.

Disconnect Your Food from Your Emotions

We've all heard about comfort foods, but different people have different comfort foods because they are attached to a particularly happy time or event from the past. Remember when I talked in the previous chapter about passing the hamburger restaurant and being seduced by the aroma of that burger and fries that your subconscious associates with a pleasurable experience from your childhood? Subconsciously, when we are feeling sad or stressed, we crave the foods that we connect with feeling happy. Sometimes we just connect food in general with happiness.

Ellen, a client of mine, told me, "Dinner was the only time for our family to be together. All day we were busy, and every night we rejoiced with food. With each mouthful and each chew, I was enjoying my family time. I wanted it to last forever, so I went on eating and eating." By bringing that memory to consciousness, Ellen was able to understand that it was really the happy memory of spending time with her family that she cherished, not the food itself.

Think about the foods that "trigger" you to overeat. It may well be that they are precisely the foods you connect with particularly pleasurable moments in the past. If you focus on remembering what those moments were, you'll be able to disconnect the emotion from the food and become more mindful of why and what you are eating. Doing a meditation to clear and focus your mind will help you to bring those subconscious associations to consciousness.

Why the Plan Works

- The "good" carbs will stabilize your blood sugar and insulin levels so that you no longer crave sugary, starchy carbs.
- The protein will fill you up and keep you feeling fuller longer so that you aren't tempted to overeat at your next meal. Protein also helps build the muscle that will boost your metabolism so that you burn calories faster.
- Your body is extremely efficient about turning the fat you eat into body fat. It takes much more energy to convert carbohydrates and protein into fat. Reducing your fat intake means that your body will have less fat to store and will burn the fat you already have much more quickly.
- Eating five times a day means that you'll be consuming fewer calories at each meal (between 300 and 500, depending on your weight and energy requirements).
- You'll never be hungry, so you won't be tempted to overeat. In fact, if you eat more than the recommended amounts, you'll find that you feel stuffed and uncomfortable.

A Gourmet Mind-Over-Body Day

My good friend Cary Neff, author of *Conscious Cuisine* and the original chef at Miraval spa, has kindly given me three recipes, to which I have added my own two "snacks" (meals 2 and 4) as a way to show how well you can eat on the 40/40/20 × 5 Fat-Loss Plan.

MEAL 1

Vegetable Omelet

Makes 1 serving

Olive oil spray
¼ cup diced mushrooms
¼ cup diced red bell pepper
1 tablespoon finely chopped red onion
4 egg whites, lightly beaten
⅛ teaspoon sea salt
⅛ teaspoon freshly ground black pepper
2 tablespoons salsa
1 tablespoon shredded low-fat Cheddar cheese
1 slice sprouted-wheat toast

Preheat the broiler.

Heat an ovenproof sauté pan over medium heat and spray it with the olive oil. Add the mushrooms and vegetables and sauté until they begin to sweat, about 5 minutes. Add the egg whites and season with the salt and pepper. Cook until the bottom and sides of the eggs are firm, about 4 minutes. Top with the salsa and shredded cheese.

Transfer the pan to the broiler for about 2 minutes, until the top of the eggs have cooked.

Flip the omelet onto a plate and serve with the toast.

Per Serving (including toast): Calories 200; Protein 20g; Total Fat 4g; Saturated Fat 1g; Carbohydrates 20g; Dietary Fiber 3g; Cholesterol 0mg; Sodium 830mg

MEAL 2

Nordine's Power Punch

If the recipe contains too much carbohydrate for you, you can eliminate the banana.

Makes 1 serving

2 tablespoons soy or whey protein powder
½ cup fat-free milk
½ cup fat-free plain yogurt
½ cup fresh strawberries
½ medium ripe banana
1 ½ cups ice cubes

Combine all the ingredients in a blender and process until smooth. Serve in a tall glass.

Per Serving: Calories 260; Protein 16g; Total Fat 1.5g; Saturated Fat 0g; Carbohydrates 51g; Dietary Fiber 5g; Cholesterol 5mg; Sodium 190mg

MEAL 3

Citrus-Dill Albacore Tuna Salad

Makes 1 serving

4 ounces water-packed albacore white tuna, drained

¼ cup chopped broccoli florets

1 tablespoon finely chopped red onion

1 tablespoon unsweetened orange juice

1 tablespoon fresh lime juice

2 teaspoons fresh lemon juice

¾ teaspoon extra virgin olive oil

⅛ teaspoon fresh dill weed

Pinch of sea salt

Pinch of freshly ground black pepper

2 leaves romaine lettuce

1 slice whole grain bread

2 slices tomato

Combine the tuna, broccoli, onion, juices, oil, dill, salt, and pepper in a bowl. Arrange the lettuce leaves on the bread, top with the tuna and then the tomato, and serve.

Per Serving: Calories 270; Protein 30g; Total Fat 8g; Saturated Fat 1.5g; Carbohydrates 22g; Dietary Fiber 7g; Cholesterol 50mg; Sodium 810mg

MEAL 4

1 cup fat-free cottage cheese
1 handful of raw, unsalted almonds (about 7 nuts)

Per Serving: Calories 220; Protein 26g; Total Fat 5g; Saturated Fat 0g; Carbohydrates 18g; Dietary Fiber 1g; Cholesterol 5 mg; Sodium 640mg

MEAL 5

Eggplant, Mushroom, and Chicken Parmesan Bake

Makes 2 servings

6 ounces skinless, boneless chicken breast
Cooking spray
4 slices (½-inch-thick) peeled eggplant
6 tablespoons organic tomato-basil pasta sauce
1 small portobello mushroom, cut into thirds
2 tablespoons fat-free ricotta cheese
¼ cup freshly grated Parmesan cheese
1 cup cooked spiral whole wheat pasta

Preheat the oven to 350 degrees.

Pound the chicken breast to ⅛ inch thick and cut it in half.

Lightly coat the bottom of a small baking pan with cooking spray. Place 2 eggplant slices in the pan. Spread with 1 tablespoon of the sauce. Top with the mushroom. Add another tablespoon of sauce, the chicken, and the ricotta. Top with the remaining eggplant slices and 1 more tablespoon sauce. Sprinkle with the grated Parmesan and bake, covered, for 20 minutes. Uncover and bake for 5 minutes longer, or until the eggplant is softened and the chicken is cooked through.

Toss the warm pasta with the remaining 3 tablespoons sauce.

Serve the Parmesan bake with the pasta on the side.

Per Serving: Calories 295; Protein 32g; Total Fat 5g; Saturated Fat 3g; Carbohydrates 30g; Dietary Fiber 5g; Cholesterol 60mg; Sodium 370mg

Do You Need to Take Vitamins with This Plan?

Although the 40/40/20 × 5 Fat-Loss Plan provides all the vitamins and minerals you need, it's my belief that taking a good-quality vitamin and mineral supplement daily can be good insurance. Look for a multivitamin with minerals that provides 100 percent of the recommended daily allowance of each one it contains.

Can Lack of Sleep Make You Fat?

At least two significant studies have shown that the less sleep you get, the more likely you are to be overweight.

Dr. Steven Heymsfield, of Columbia University and St. Luke's–Roosevelt Hospital in New York, and James Gangwisch, a Columbia University epidemiologist, headed a study that looked at the information provided by 18,000 adults who participated in the federal government's National Health and Nutrition Survey throughout the 1980s. The researchers found that people who got less than four hours of sleep a night were 73 percent more likely to be obese than those who got the recommended seven to nine hours of sleep. Those who averaged five hours of sleep had a 50 percent greater risk of obesity, and those who got six hours had a 23 percent greater risk.

In another study, researchers at Stanford University and the University of Wisconsin–Madison looked at more than 1,000 participants in the Wisconsin Sleep Cohort Study who spent a night in the lab and then had a blood sample taken upon waking. The researchers discovered that those who slept shorter times had higher blood levels of ghrelin, a hormone that increases appetite, and lower levels of leptin, a hormone that decreases appetite. The shorter sleepers also had a higher body mass index.

The long and the short of it would seem to be, get a good night's sleep!

Can You Drink Alcohol on This Plan?

I believe that drinking a glass of wine (but no more than that) with your evening meal can be an enjoyable component of this or any healthy lifestyle. Too much alcohol, however, can adversely affect both your health and your weight. Remember that a four-ounce glass of wine or one ounce of almost any hard liquor contains 100 calories, and if you have a mixed drink, you'll be consuming even more calories. Additionally, alcohol is dehydrating, so it's wise to have a glass of water for every glass of alcohol you drink.

What Happens If You Cheat?

Actually, I recommend that you cheat, but only at specific intervals and never for more than a day. I'm sure you remember that when we talked about determining your core desire, I advised you to concentrate on how you would feel when you had achieved your goal. If you need to lose thirty pounds or more, that goal can seem overwhelming at first. Therefore, I suggest that you focus instead on losing a few pounds at a time, and each time you achieve that small victory, I want you to celebrate with a "cheat day."

A cheat day accomplishes two things: It prevents you from feeling deprived, and it helps boost your metabolism so that you'll burn more calories when you return to the plan. You'll probably gain a couple of pounds on your cheat day, but they will likely disappear within seventy-two hours.

- Set your mind on losing two to five pounds in the next two weeks. (The heavier you are, the more weight you can expect to lose.)
- At the end of the two-week period, celebrate your victory with a cheat day.
- Reset your goal as soon as you finish celebrating.

Clients who use this method of self-motivation to achieve their long-term goals report that they no longer "dread" the idea of having to lose weight but actually enjoy the process. One woman told me that after she'd lost 110 pounds, she felt and looked fantastic and wanted to keep losing more. When I asked her why, she said, "I enjoy the process and the cheat days—especially the cheat days."

To Weigh or Not to Weigh, That Is the Question

Some people become stressed just from thinking of getting on a scale, while others weigh themselves obsessively. I strongly suggest that you try to find a happy medium.

You'll know if you're losing weight just by looking in the mirror and feeling your clothes getting looser, but I recommend that you weigh yourself once a week as a way to keep track of your progress. That way, you'll know when you've achieved each small goal and can celebrate with a cheat day. But don't weigh yourself more often than that, because the scale can be misleading. Everyone experiences weight fluctuations from day to day, and these may cause you to become discouraged for no reason.

When you do weigh yourself, using a balance scale rather than a spring scale will give you a more accurate result. I also recommend that you always weigh yourself at the same time of day, preferably first thing in the morning, before you've had anything to eat—which is obviously when you'll weigh the least. More important, if you weigh yourself at the end of the day, the results will be less consistent because you won't be eating exactly the same thing every day.

One caveat: As you begin to lose fat and gain muscle tone, the number on the scale may not be an accurate representation of your progress. During the first month or so, you may actually weigh more even though you look better. That initial weight gain will reverse itself in a few weeks.

Reach Your Peak of Fitness One Small Step at a Time

The people who conquer Mount Everest or Mount Kilimanjaro get to the summit one small step at a time. They climb and they rest, climb and rest, celebrating each new plateau along the way. And when they get to the top, they are rewarded with a limitless vista and a belief in their ability to achieve virtually anything.

As you embark on your own journey to the peak of fitness, I want you to do the same.

- As you set out, celebrate the fact that you've been able to harness your mind to change your body by discovering your core desire and setting your intention to achieve it.
- Celebrate each step you take toward your goal by looking at your list of affirmations and reminding yourself that you have within you everything it takes to achieve whatever you desire.
- If you come to a rough patch and feel that you may falter, take time to visualize again what it will feel like when you get there. Just doing that will help calm the anxiety that naturally occurs when you are trying to change and replace it with the positive energy you need to go on.
- Know that you, too, can and will reach the peak and revel in what you've achieved.

In the following chapter, I'll give you the final tool you need to achieve the body you've always dreamed of having. You already have what you need to nourish yourself mentally and physically. Now you need to add the all-important exercise component, which will help increase your metabolism so that you lose weight faster while also building muscle and losing fat. Like the 40/40/20 × 5 Fat-Loss Plan, it's easy to follow and designed to fit into even the busiest schedule. And remember that doing this for yourself is something you need to achieve your core desire.

Six

The 12/12 × 5 Ultimate Workout Plan

If you look in the mirror and you don't want the body you see, you will actually be attracting more of what you don't want. If you want a great body, you need to think about having a great body.

When we left Amanda in the previous chapter, she had shifted her perspective so that she was able to see her fitness goal in terms of achieving maximum health. When I began working with her to design an exercise program to go with her new approach to nutrition, I discovered that what she'd been doing before coming to see me was to concentrate on aerobic exercise for ninety minutes a day, seven days a week, while she spent only one session a week on strength training.

Amanda had been obsessed with the elliptical cross-trainer to the point where one day she was on it for so long that it actually rebelled by blowing a fuse. But Amanda is far from unique in her obsession with cardio training. Go to any large gym any day of the week, and you'll find the cardio machines occupied by people who are there when you begin your workout and still there when you finish.

What I was able to teach Amanda is exactly what I'll be teaching you in this chapter: spending hours on the cross-trainer, treadmill, or stair-climber will never get you in shape. You need to do a combination of strength and cardiovascular training, for a reasonable amount of time, and your strength training always needs to precede the cardio segment of your workout.

Shift Your Perspective on Fitness

What I'm asking you to do in this book is no different from what I asked of Amanda. I want you to consider fitness from a new perspective. Instead of mere body consciousness, I'm asking you to approach fitness from the point of view of mind and body consciousness. This is what I call mindful fitness. It is the only way to achieve what you truly desire.

If you go to the gym and turn off your brain while your body performs a routine, you'll be gaining only half the benefit of what you're doing. Being aware of where you are and what you're doing at every moment means that you are not only concentrating on the exercise being performed but also remembering the purpose of doing it. Perform every movement and every set of every exercise as if your life depended on it. By remaining mindful of what you're doing and why you're doing it, you will be not only goal-oriented but also process-oriented; in other words, you'll be moving from "doing" to "being." So the most important thing you can do for your body as you begin the exercise program in this chapter is to keep your mind present and focused. Since your body takes its instructions from your mind, a lack of focus results in a lack of effectiveness. And when you make each moment of your workout mindful, you have to spend less time in the gym because you're getting more out of every exercise.

Seek Quality, Not Quantity

One of the first questions clients ask me is, "How much exercise is enough?" And my answer is always the same: "Spending more time working out is not necessarily better." The key is to do the right routine with the right amount of focus and intensity. That ought to be really good news if you've been using the number one excuse for not exercising: "I don't have enough time!"

When it comes to exercise, there's a scientific reason why more isn't necessarily better. Cortisol is used by the body to break down muscle protein for energy, and cortisol levels begin to rise after about an hour of training. Since you don't want to break down muscle tissue and you don't want to stress your body by raising your cortisol levels, you shouldn't work out for more than an hour at a time.

In addition, research has shown that working at greater intensity for a shorter period of time is more beneficial for fat loss than working at lower intensity for a longer time.

Throughout my career as a professional athlete, I never worked my body for more than an hour a day, and even then I split my workout into two 30-minute sessions. The program I'm offering you here requires only 24 minutes a day, 5 days a week, of focused and effective exercise.

The purpose of the 12/12 × 5 Ultimate Workout Plan is to keep yourself moving by taking only short breaks between exercises. You'll be working your body aerobically while still challenging your strength, which will maximize fat loss and increase muscle tone. You could spend a lot more time in the gym chatting and socializing, but that would only make your workout less rather than more effective.

How Does It Work?

Like my nutrition plan, it's as easy as 1, 2, 3!

- Do 12 minutes of upper body (chest, back, shoulders, triceps, biceps, upper abs, and waist) strength training *followed by* 12 minutes of cardio training on days 1 and 4.
- Do 12 minutes of lower body (quads, glutes, hamstrings, adductors, abductors, calves, lower abs, and waist) strength training *followed by* 12 minutes of cardio training on days 2 and 5.
- Do 24 minutes of cardio training only on day 3.

Here's what your 12/12 × 5 workout week will look like.

Day 1: 12 minutes upper body strength training + 12 minutes cardio training

Day 2: 12 minutes lower body strength training + 12 minutes cardio training

Day 3: 24 minutes cardio training only

Day 4: 12 minutes upper body strength training + 12 minutes cardio training

Day 5: 12 minutes lower body strength training + 12 minutes cardio training

Days 6 and 7: Rest!

Specific strength training exercises for each day and each muscle group begin on page 140.

Be Mindful Before You Begin

One of the most effective tools I can give you for getting the most out of your exercise program is to do what I always did when I was training for competition. Before you begin each session, visualize each movement. Actually see your joints moving and your muscles working. See yourself completing the session with perfect form. By doing that, you are imprinting the movements on your subconscious, and your body will seek to replicate what you have created in your mind.

Now visualize how you will look when you've achieved the body you want to have. See your muscles chiseled and strong. See your waistline slim. Concentrate on your success in order to create the same sense of excitement and the energy you felt when you first discovered your true core desire.

The next 24 minutes are going to be all about you, so begin by focusing positively on yourself.

Warm Up Your Body Along with Your Mind

Just as you "warm up" your mind with visualizations before you begin to work out, you need to warm up your muscles so that they're prepared to perform the tasks you'll be asking of them. You can do this by walking in place while swinging your arms or, if you're in a gym, using any cardio machine, such as a treadmill, set at a moderate pace for 5 minutes.

Warming up allows your heart rate to increase gradually and produces the blood flow required by your muscles during exercise. Working out without a proper warm-up can lead to unnecessary injuries.

STRENGTH TRAINING ALWAYS COMES FIRST

You may be wondering why your strength training always comes *before* your cardio training. That's because to achieve maximum results, you need to have your greatest strength and energy to do your strength training. In addition, the strength training will empty your glycogen stores (the storage form of glucose) so that you begin to burn fat more quickly when you start your cardio exercise. It's important that you stick to this sequence if you want to get the most out of your workouts.

What You Need to Know About Strength Training

Simply put, strength training means working out with weights or machines that offer resistance in order to strengthen and build your bones and muscles. This is possibly the single most important thing you can do to improve your health and increase longevity.

After the age of thirty, everyone starts to lose both bone and muscle mass. Strength training can help to rebuild lost bone and decrease the risk of osteoporosis, which strikes half of all women over the age of fifty and can affect men as well. In addition, the American College of Sports Medicine has found that lean muscle mass decreases by almost 50 percent between the ages of twenty and ninety. And whenever we lose lean muscle, we replace it with fat.

Strength training will not only help to keep you healthy; it also will help you to lose weight. One reason for this is that muscle burns more calories than fat, so the more muscle you build, the faster you'll burn calories. But there's more. Recent research at Colorado State University indicates that after you've completed a strength training workout, your metabolism remains elevated for several hours, which means that you're burning more calories not only during your workout but also for a long time after you finish.

Any strength training program should target all the major muscle groups in the legs, chest, back, shoulders, and arms, as well as—especially for women—the core muscles in the abdomen and lower back. Strengthening the abdomen and lower back helps to develop bone in the hips and promotes good posture, which makes it easier to perform the activities of daily life with more strength and better balance.

Will Strength Training Turn You Into the Hulk?

Traditionally, women (except professional athletes) have stayed away from strength training because they were afraid of developing too much muscle. Luckily, that trend has been changing over the past few years because women often have the most to gain in terms of health benefits from their strength training workouts.

So here are the facts:

- No one, man or woman, will bulk up from a well-designed strength training program.
- Bodybuilders typically train for several hours a day over the course of several years while consuming huge amounts of calories. When I was training as a professional athlete, I ate more than 4000 calories a day, and some bodybuilders I know eat more than 7000!
- Strength training helps to combat a variety of diseases—particularly those associated with aging—and to alleviate the adverse effects of stress.

Before You Begin Strength Training, Gauge Your Level of Intensity

You should be able to perform at least 12 repetitions of each exercise, with the last 3 requiring a challenging effort. If you can't do 12, you may be using too much weight. If you can do more than 15 without feeling challenged, the weight is probably too light. Test yourself and adjust your weight accordingly.

Your strength may begin to improve after just three to four weeks of consistent training. When you no longer feel that your weight sets are challenging enough, you will need to increase the amount of weight you are using to continue those gains.

Free Weights or Machines—Which Way Is Better?

I'm certainly not against using machines for strength training. In fact, I continue to use them as part of my own strength training workout. That said, for most people who are not professional athletes, free weights are more compatible with the tasks we perform every day. Groceries, books, furniture, home-care tools, and children—in other words the things we lift and move in the course of daily life—are not fixed weights that move in only one fixed direction. We pick up and move these items without the benefit of guides, rails, and levers. Therefore, we need to train our bodies to move in multiple planes and angles to comply with real-life movements. Free weights—dumbbells, medicine balls, and ankle weights—are better training tools than machines for everyday life, not only because they mimic our most common movements but also because they help us develop better balance and strengthen the muscles of the torso that stabilize the spine and provide a solid foundation for movement in the extremities.

In addition, during the first four to six weeks of strength training, you're increasing muscular coordination and sensory awareness, both of which develop less quickly if you use machines that work in only one plane of motion. So even if you decide to use machines, I recommend that you begin your training with free weights.

The Ten Commandments of Mindful Strength Training

Keeping these ten dos and don'ts in mind will ensure that you gain the maximum benefit from each and every workout.

1. **Warm up.** A 5-minute warm-up will bring more blood to your muscles, lubricate your joints, and prevent unnecessary injury.

2. **Stretch.** Stretching between sets of strength exercises will not only make you more flexible and increase your range of motion, but it will also increase blood flow to your muscles and break down the buildup of lactic acid that can make you stiff and sore. When you lift weights, your body changes glucose into ATP (adenosine triphosphate) to fuel your performance. During this process, lactic acid quickly builds up in your muscles. When it increases past a certain point,

you feel an intense burning sensation. I recommend an appropriate stretch for each muscle group beginning on page 164.

3. **Focus.** Concentrate on every move you perform. Forget about paying your bills, making your grocery list, or preparing for your next meeting. When your mind wanders, bring it back by becoming aware of your breathing and what your muscles are doing. When you stay in the moment, you will be connected to the muscle you are working, your range of motion will increase, and the quality of your workout will be magnified. To help you do that, I suggest that you stare at a fixed spot within your direct line of vision, because when your eyes are moving, you are more likely to be distracted.

4. **Maintain proper sequencing.** Proper sequencing of your exercises is important for improving strength and muscle tone. Go from large muscles to small, from multiple-joint to single-joint exercises, from higher to lower intensity. I have organized the exercises in this book in the order you should perform them.

5. **Maintain speed and form.** Each exercise can be broken down into two segments, the positive and the negative. In a bench press, for example, pushing the weight from your chest toward the ceiling is the positive; lowering it is the negative. Always perform your movements with mindfulness and control. Don't rush or jerk the weights. A good, challenging set consists of 12 to 15 repetitions done with controlled speed and perfect form using the full range of motion. If you can't do that, you're probably using too much weight.

6. **Progress.** Add more weight to each exercise as you gain strength so that you are always using the greatest amount of weight possible without compromising your form.

7. **Challenge your set.** Take your set to the point where you can't perform another repetition without compromising form and/or speed.

8. **Breathe properly.** Proper breathing during strength training is exactly the opposite of what it should be when you're stretching. During strength training, exhale through your mouth as you complete the positive segment of the exercise and inhale on the negative. I tell my clients to count their reps aloud (if you're in

a public place, just whisper) as they breathe until the breathing process becomes automatic and natural.

9. **Rest.** To maintain proper intensity, you should rest for no more than 30 seconds between sets or exercises. This is all the time it takes to stretch, change weights, and prepare for the next set or exercise.

10. **Give your muscles time to recover.** You should never work the same muscle groups two days in a row. That's why this plan alternates upper and lower body exercises.

Expect to Feel It the Next Day

If you haven't exercised in a while, or if you're changing the way you exercise (so that you're using different muscles), it's normal to feel some muscle soreness within the next twelve to forty-eight hours. You may also feel some muscle fatigue, stiffness, or weakness. Don't worry about it. As your muscles adapt to the new stress, they'll grow stronger, and the soreness will be a thing of the past. Meanwhile, if you're feeling sore, treat yourself to a nice, relaxing, hot bath—it's better for your mind and your body than ibuprofen any day.

Get the Most from Your Cardio Training

Cardiovascular training is defined by its ability to elevate your heart rate, which strengthens the heart muscle so that it circulates blood more efficiently and delivers fresh oxygen to the muscles and organs.

Clearly, anything that's good for your heart is good for your overall health and longevity, and cardio fitness is a defense against heart disease. But that isn't all. If you've ever experienced the endorphin rush that follows a good cardio workout, you know that there's nothing more exhilarating. It can literally lift the dark curtain of depression by delivering the right neurotransmitters to the cells.

Because you've just finished your strength training exercises, your heart rate will already be elevated and you'll be warmed up when you start the cardio part of your routine. The key is to raise your heart rate enough and to keep it elevated for long enough to achieve the maximum benefit. To do this, you can use whatever type of cardio equipment you prefer—treadmill, bike, stair-climber, elliptical trainer, or cross-trainer; you can take an aerobics class; or you can simply walk, jog, or run.

How Do You Know If You're Working Hard Enough to Raise Your Heart Rate?

Because different people may have different resting heart rates or may find it difficult to take their own heart rate, I recommend a scale based on your rate of perceived exertion, or RPE, to help you determine the intensity of your cardio training.

Your exercise should be enjoyable, stimulating, and energizing so that you actually look forward to it rather than dreading it. Working too hard is one of the primary reasons people stop exercising altogether. That said, you don't want to be wasting your time by doing too little, because if you don't begin seeing results, that also might lead to your giving up.

My cardio program is based on interval training, which means that you do 2 to 3 minutes at moderate intensity (such as walking) followed by 2 to 3 minutes at relatively high intensity (jogging, running, or walking at an incline, for example). Your moderate intervals should be at a 3 or 4 on the RPE scale; your high-intensity intervals should be at an 8 or 9. I don't recommend that you ever go beyond a 9.

If you've been sedentary up to this point, I recommend that you keep your intensity levels between 3 and 6. You can then increase them as you build strength and endurance.

Here's an easy-to-use RPE scale.

RPE 1 and 2   Very easy; you can carry on a conversation with no effort.
RPE 3   Easy; you can carry on a conversation with almost no effort.
RPE 4   Moderately easy; you can talk with minimal effort.
RPE 5   Moderate; talking requires some effort.
RPE 6   Moderately difficult; talking requires quite a bit of effort.
RPE 7   Difficult; conversation requires a lot of effort.
RPE 8   Very difficult; conversation requires maximum effort.
RPE 9 and 10   Maximum effort; conversation is impossible. (Don't worry about whether you've made it all the way to 10. In fact, don't even try. When you can't carry on a conversation, you've reached your limit.)

Stop exercising immediately if you feel any of the following:

- Chest discomfort such as pressure or burning
- Chest discomfort radiating to the shoulders or down the arm
- Extreme dizziness, weakness, or disorientation
- Extreme shortness of breath or difficulty breathing

At Home or in the Gym?

Since 25 percent of your brain is involved with visual processing, it makes sense to me that seeing people who look the way you want to look will make you want to work harder. That means choosing a gym where people go to work out, not to stand around and socialize. This is my formula for success:

A positive mental attitude + a positive environment + a positive support system = rapid results

Going to the gym with the right attitude, choosing a gym where you're surrounded by other motivated people, and finding a workout partner or coach who will support your efforts is the way to achieve the most in the least amount of time.

If you think you'd prefer to work out at home, you need to be sure that you'll remain motivated, that you'll be free from distractions, and that you have the proper equipment. Unless you live in a climate where you can engage in outdoor activities year-round, machines will make your exercise routine a lot easier and more convenient. They also add variety, which may help to keep you challenged and interested. Although the exercises in this book don't require a great deal of equipment, the cardio machines available in a gym will give you a lot more variety and flexibility than what you'll have at home. In addition, a 1999 market intelligence report by Kalorama Information showed that 80 percent of home exercise equipment is not used after the first year.

My own favorite piece of equipment is the elliptical cross-trainer, which provides a workout for both your upper and lower body. I also like the elliptical trainer and the treadmill, both of which provide a good, hard lower body workout. Stationary bikes and stair-climbers don't work you as hard, but you can certainly get a better workout on a stationary bike set at a high intensity than you would on an elliptical cross-trainer set at a low intensity. Elliptical cross-trainers and elliptical trainers also put less stress on your joints than, for example, a treadmill, because they are nonimpact machines. The bottom line is to use the machine, so pick the one you like best or change things up if that's what keeps you going.

I believe that making an appointment (even if it's only with yourself) to be somewhere and do something at a specific time can be a powerful motivator. In this regard, I think that you're better off going to a gym, if possible.

Interval Training: The Ultimate Cardio Workout

Interval training is my favorite way to burn fat. It means changing the level of intensity at which you're working out every 2 to 3 minutes, which allows you to push yourself harder than if you were working at a higher level of intensity for a longer period of time.

During your 12-minute cardio workout, try jogging or walking at your normal pace for 2 to 3 minutes, then increase your pace for the next 2 to 3 minutes before slowing down again. Or if you're on a stationary bicycle, pedal at a normal pace for 2 to 3 minutes, then increase the resistance for 2 to 3 minutes, and so on. Always start at low intensity. You can build up the speed or resistance of your intervals so that with each high-intensity segment, you'll be working yourself harder than you did the previous time. For example:

- Work at an RPE of 5 for 2 minutes. (You should already by warmed up to this level after your strength training.)
- Increase to an RPE of 6 for the next 2 minutes.
- Slow down to an RPE of 5 for 2 minutes.
- Increase to an RPE of 7 for the next 2 minutes.
- Cool down with 4 minutes at an RPE of 3.

That's your total 12 minutes.

To increase your RPE:

- On a treadmill: Increase or decrease the incline, or increase or decrease the speed.
- On an elliptical trainer or elliptical cross-trainer: Increase or decrease the resistance.
- On an upright or recumbent stationary bicycle: Increase or decrease the speed, or increase or decrease the resistance.

- On a stair-climber: Increase or decrease the speed, or increase or decrease the resistance.
- On a rowing machine: Increase or decrease the resistance.

After Your Workout, Take Time to Cool Down

Cooling down is as important as warming up because it allows your heart rate and breathing to return gradually to normal levels. Otherwise, you might experience the dizziness that results from blood pooling in the large muscles of the legs when vigorous activity is stopped too abruptly. That's why I ask you to finish your cardio workout at an RPE of 3 for the last 4 minutes.

STRENGTH TRAINING EXERCISES

Remember to warm up for 5 minutes before you begin.
You will be doing 2 sets of each exercise:

- 1 set of 15 repetitions with moderate weight
- 1 set of 12 repetitions with heavier weight

The only exception to this is the abdominal exercises, for which you need to do 20 to 30 repetitions.

The last 3 repetitions of each set should require a challenging effort if the weight is correct. As you gain strength and your sets no longer seem as challenging, increase the weight for the first set by 5 to 10 pounds.

Do the appropriate stretch for 15 seconds and rest for 15 seconds between sets. The stretches that are appropriate for each muscle group are found on pages 164–169.

Remember that day 3 is for cardio training only and days 6 and 7 are for rest.

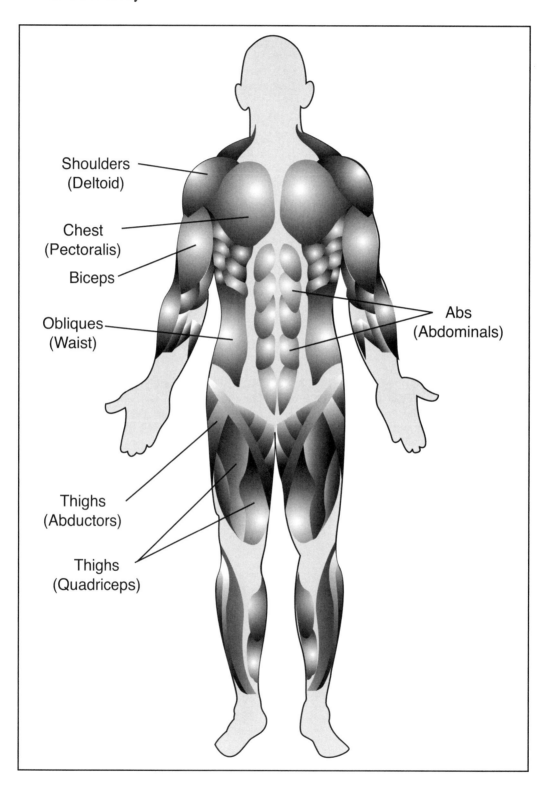

Shoulders
(Deltoid)

Chest
(Pectoralis)

Biceps

Obliques
(Waist)

Abs
(Abdominals)

Thighs
(Abductors)

Thighs
(Quadriceps)

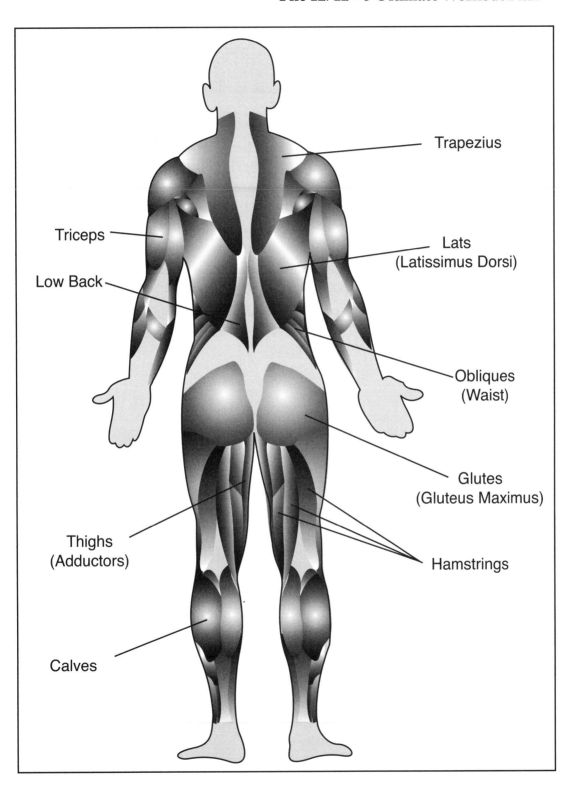

Trapezius

Triceps

Lats
(Latissimus Dorsi)

Low Back

Obliques
(Waist)

Glutes
(Gluteus Maximus)

Thighs
(Adductors)

Hamstrings

Calves

ABDOMINALS

Bent-Knee Abdominal Crunch

Strengthens and tones the stomach muscles

Lie on a mat on the floor with your arms behind your head, knees bent, and feet flat on the floor. Contract your abdominals as you raise your shoulders and upper back toward the ceiling. Keep your head and neck in line with your spine. Keep your lower and middle back on the floor. Return to your starting position.

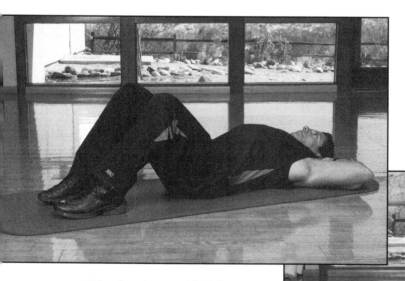

Nordine's Mindful Tip: This exercise is working your upper abdominals. Avoid lifting the rest of your body off the floor and pulling your neck forward with your hands, which could stress your neck muscles.

CHEST

Dumbbell Incline Press

Great for developing and lifting your upper chest muscles

Lying on your back on a bench set at a 45-degree incline, hold a dumbbell in each hand with your arms bent and your hands at either side of your chest. Press both dumbbells straight up with your palms facing inward. Once your arms are fully extended, gently tap the dumbbells together before slowly returning them to the starting position.

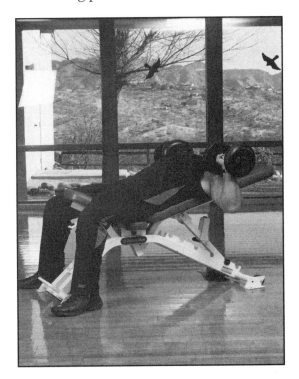
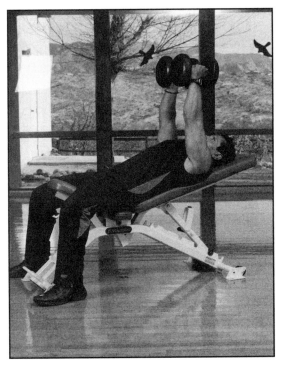

Nordine's Mindful Tip: Keep your neck and shoulders relaxed and avoid arching your back while pressing the weight, as this can stress your lower back. Make sure the bench is at no more than a 45-degree angle; otherwise you will be working your shoulders instead of your chest muscles.

LATS

Single-Arm Bent-Over Dumbbell Row

Great for your upper back

Kneel with your right knee on a bench and your left foot on the floor. Holding a dumbbell in your left hand, pull the dumbbell back until your upper arm is just beyond horizontal or at the height of your back. Lower the dumbbell until your arm is extended and your shoulder is stretched. Complete the set, then change sides and repeat the exercise.

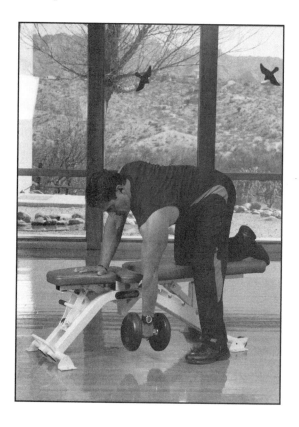
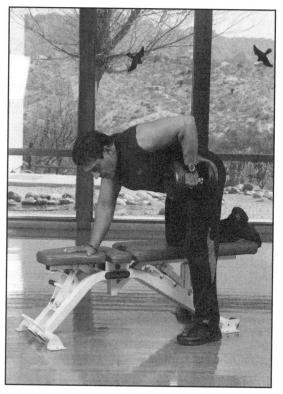

Nordine's Mindful Tip: Avoid hunching or rounding your back. Keep your neck aligned with the rest of your body by looking down at all times.

SHOULDERS

Seated Dumbbell Press

Good for toning the shoulder muscles

Note: If you have shoulder problems or high blood pressure, you should not do this exercise.

Sit on a bench, preferably one with a backrest. Hold a dumbbell in each hand, arms bent, elbows at your sides, hands level with your ears, palms facing inward. Press the dumbbells upward until your arms are fully extended and rotate your palms forward at the end of the movement. Slowly return to the starting position.

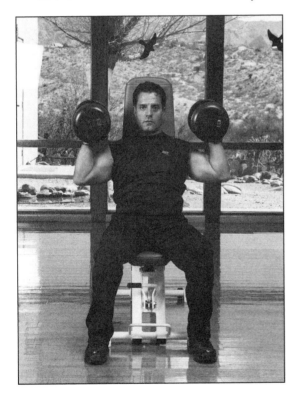 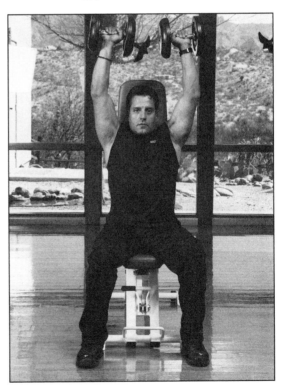

Nordine's Mindful Tip: Look straight ahead, don't hunch over, and avoid bouncing the dumbbells onto your shoulders.

BICEPS

Standing Dumbbell Curl

Works your biceps and gives you better freedom of motion than the barbell curl because your arms are not fixed in one position

With your feet shoulder-width apart and your knees slightly bent, tuck in your navel and hold the weights at your sides with your palms facing your body. Curl your arms toward your shoulders, rotating your palms upward while beginning the curl. Slowly return to the starting position.

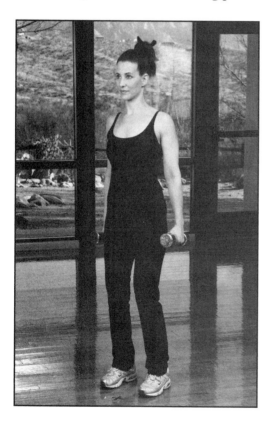 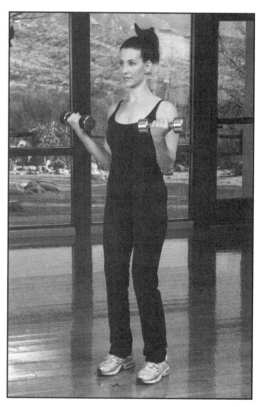

Nordine's Mindful Tip: If you have a tendency to move any part of your body other than your arms when doing this exercise, try using lighter weights.

TRICEPS

Bench Dip

Uses your own body weight to strengthen and tone your triceps

Position yourself with your back to a bench, legs out in front of you and slightly bent, hands gripping the edge of the bench, elbows close to your sides. Lower your body until you feel the full stretch, then raise yourself back up and repeat.

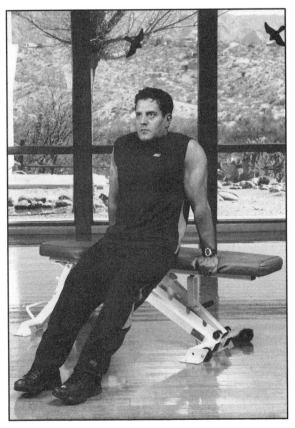 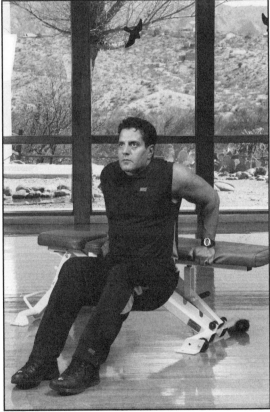

Nordine's Mindful Tip: Lift your body with love. Do not lower your body too low, as this can stress your shoulders unnecessarily. Keep your hips as close to the bench as possible.

ABDOMINALS

Trunk Twist

Great for shaping your waist

Stand holding a broom handle across the back of your shoulders, tighten your abdominal muscles, and rotate your upper body, twisting from the waist to one side and then the other.

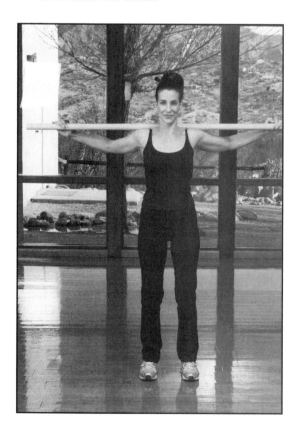 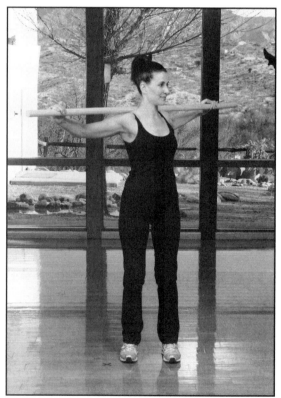

Nordine's Mindful Tip: Remember to keep your back straight as you twist. Don't hunch forward or arch backward.

THIGHS

Alternate Weighted Leg Extension (Ankle Weights)

*Shapes the front of your thighs and strengthens the muscles around the knees,
which is particularly important for runners*

Note: Do not perform this exercise if you have problems with your knees.

Sit on a flat bench and attach weights to both ankles. Grab the sides of the bench and, keeping your knees bent at a 90-degree angle, raise one foot a couple of inches off the floor. Keeping your back straight, slowly extend your leg upward until it is about parallel to the ground. Contract your thigh muscles and then return your foot to the starting position. Repeat the exercise with the opposite leg.

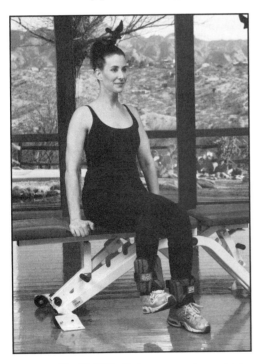 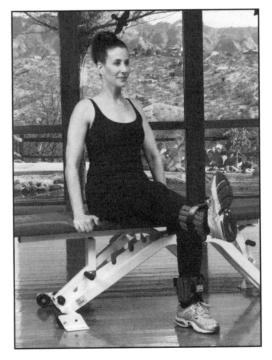

Nordine's Mindful Tip: Avoid locking your knee at full extension and do not jerk the weight on the way down.

GLUTES AND THIGHS

Dumbbell Squat

Strengthens and tones your thighs and glutes, giving you shapely buns

Stand holding the dumbbells at your sides. With your back straight, your head up and facing straight ahead, bend your knees until your thighs are parallel to the floor. Keep your abdominals tight by tucking in your navel, and keep your weight on your heels. Slowly return to a standing position by extending your knees and hips until your legs are straight.

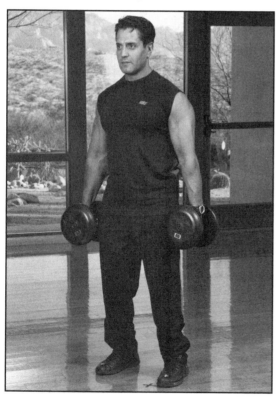 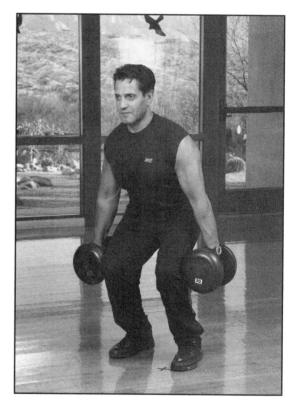

Nordine's Mindful Tip: It is important to keep your feet about shoulder-width apart and your back straight. Avoid squatting too low; keep your thighs parallel to the floor.

GLUTES AND THIGHS

Dumbbell Lunge

Excellent for shaping your glutes and thighs

Stand upright with your back straight, looking straight ahead (into a mirror if possible). With your legs shoulder-width apart, step forward, bending your front leg until your thigh is parallel to the floor. Return to your starting position. Complete the set, then change legs and repeat the exercise.

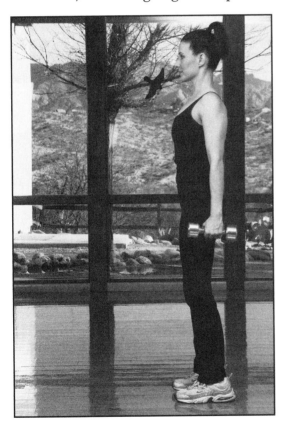
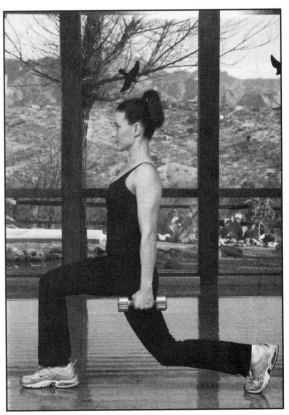

Nordine's Mindful Tip: Do not step too far out, which could put too much stress on your knees. Make sure you step down with your front foot flat on the floor.

HAMSTRINGS

Alternate Lying Leg Curl

Good for working the backs of your legs

Attach weights to your ankles and lie on your stomach on a bench. Keeping your feet flexed toward your knees, bring one heel as close to your buttocks as possible. Slowly bring your heel back to the starting position and repeat the exercise with the opposite leg.

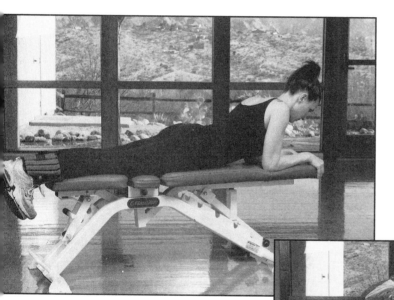

Nordine's Mindful Tip: Keep your pelvis against the bench at all times and avoid arching your back.

CALVES

Dumbbell One-Leg Standing Heel Raise

Works the outer part of your calves

Hold a dumbbell at your side with your left hand and place your right hand on a fitness bar or against a wall for support. Stand on your right foot with your toes on a two-inch-thick board or book, heel on the floor and your left knee crossed over your right. With your right knee slightly bent, rise up on your toes as high as possible. Change legs and repeat the exercise.

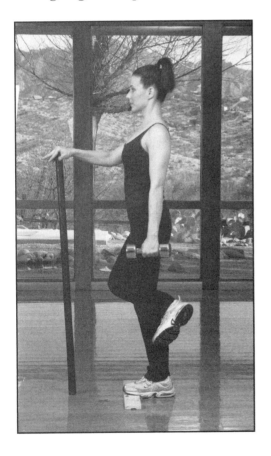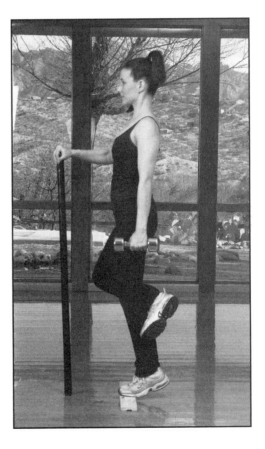

Nordine's Mindful Tip: Avoid arching your back when doing this exercise.

ABDOMINALS

Twisting Crunches

Another great exercise for your upper abs and waist

Lie on a mat with your hands behind your head, your knees bent at a 90-degree angle. Curl your upper body forward while rotating one elbow toward the opposite knee. Return to your starting position and repeat with the opposite elbow and knee.

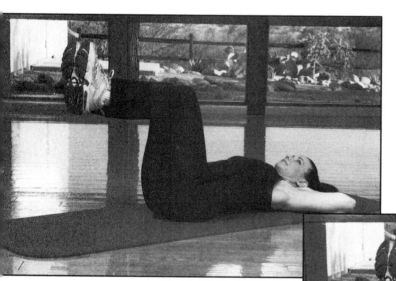

Nordine's Mindful Tip: Always keep your neck straight, not bent forward or backward, with a space between your chin and your chest. If you have a lower-back problem, bend your knees and keep your feet on the floor.

CHEST

Dumbbell Incline Fly

Works the upper and lateral area of your chest

Lie faceup on a bench set at a 45-degree angle with your feet flat on the floor. Hold a dumbbell in each hand with your arms above your head, elbows slightly bent and pointed out, hands facing each other. Turn your hands so that your palms are facing upward and lower your arms until they are parallel to the floor.

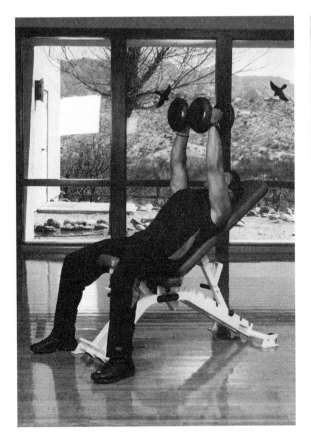
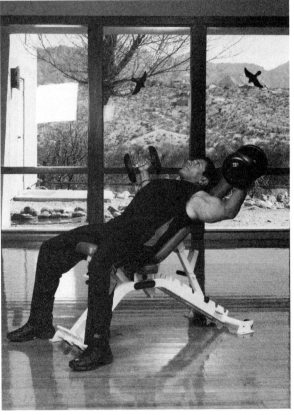

Nordine's Mindful Tip: To avoid damaging your shoulder joints, don't overstretch when lowering your arms.

LATS

Dumbbell Pull Over

A wonderful exercise for working your upper back muscles and lifting your chest to give you a more graceful appearance

Lying on a flat bench with your knees bent, grasp a dumbbell with both hands and raise it directly over your head. Keeping your arms slightly bent, slowly lower the dumbbell behind your head as far as you comfortably can. You should feel the stretch in your upper back. Contract your back muscles as you push the dumbbell back to the overhead position.

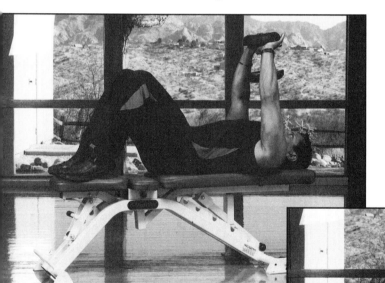

Nordine's Mindful Tip: Keep your lower back flat against the bench at all times.

SHOULDERS

Seated Bent-Over Rear Deltoid Dumbbell Raise

Great for the back of your shoulders and your upper back area

Sit at the end of a bench with your knees bent at 90 degrees, keeping your feet flat on the floor. Hold a dumbbell in each hand hanging down at your sides, and bend over at the waist. Bend your elbows slightly and raise the dumbbells up and out to the sides until they are almost parallel to the floor. Contract your rear delts (the muscles at the back of your shoulders) at the top of the movement and then slowly lower the dumbbells to the starting position.

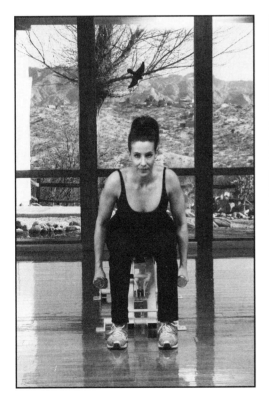 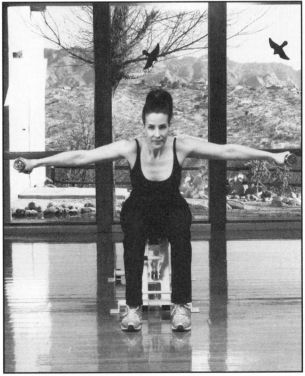

Nordine's Mindful Tip: Avoid swinging your body upward as you move your arms, as this can create unnecessary strain on your neck and back muscles.

BICEPS

Single-Arm Dumbbell Preacher Curl

Strengthens and tones the lower part of your biceps

Sit at the edge of a bench with your legs wide apart. With your right arm hanging down between your legs, grasp a dumbbell in your right hand. Brace your upper arm on the inside of your right knee and raise the dumbbell toward your shoulder. Slowly return the dumbbell to the starting position. Complete the set, then change hands and repeat the exercise.

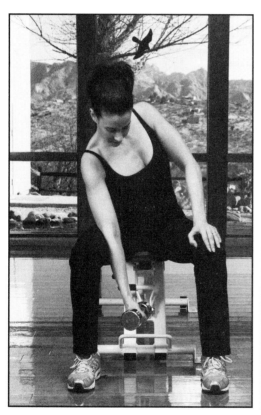 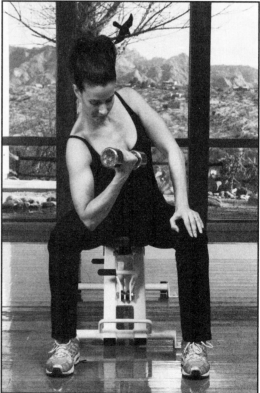

Nordine's Mindful Tip: Concentrate on your form. Perform the movement in a slow and controlled fashion.

TRICEPS
Dumbbell Triceps Kickback

Great for shaping your triceps

Place your right hand and knee on a flat bench so that you are slightly bent over. Your left foot should be flat on the floor, with your leg slightly forward to secure your lower back. Hold a dumbbell in your left hand, with your elbow bent and high. Straighten your arm back until it is fully extended. Slowly return the dumbbell to the starting position. Complete the set, then change sides and repeat the exercise.

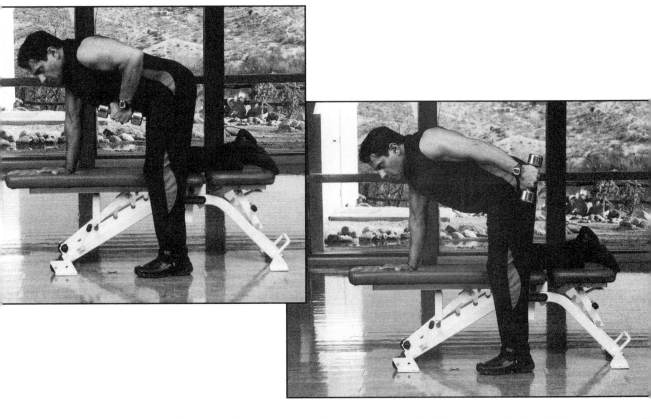

Nordine's Mindful Tip: Keep your elbow against your side. Keep your body still and parallel to the floor at all times. Avoid hunching your back.

Day 5: Lower Body

ABDOMINALS

Reverse Crunch

Great for your lower abdominals

Lie on a mat, arms at your sides and palms flat on the floor. Bend your knees at a 90-degree angle. Now contract your abdominals and curl your hips up until your lower back clears the floor. Return to your starting position and repeat.

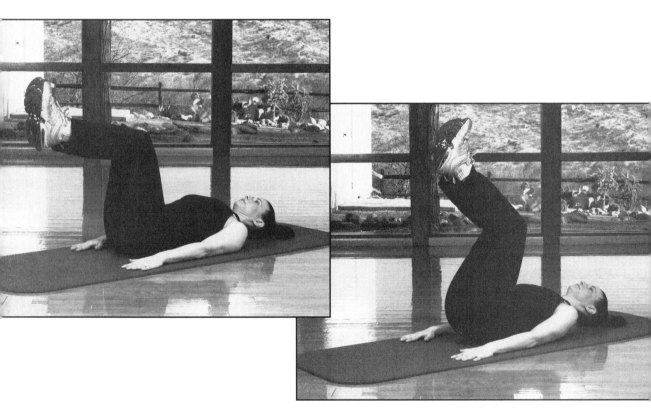

Nordine's Mindful Tip: Remember to keep your knees bent at a 90-degree angle. Avoid bringing your legs too close to your body.

GLUTES AND THIGHS

Dumbbell Step Up

Tightens your buns and shapes your thighs

Stand in front of a solid box holding your dumbbells at your sides. Keeping your head up and your back straight, step onto the box with one foot and bring your other leg up toward your chest. Complete the set and repeat with the opposite leg.

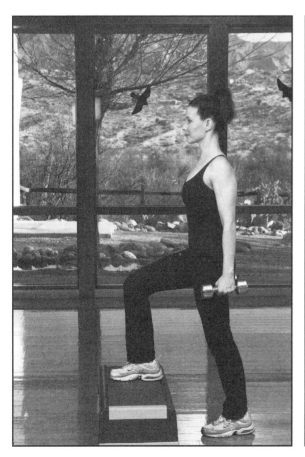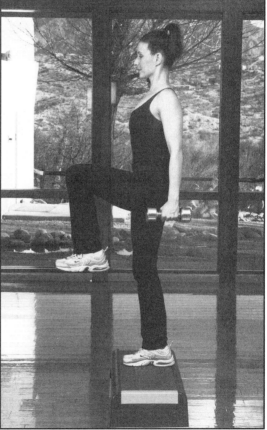

Nordine's Mindful Tip: Keep your torso straight while you do the exercise. Standing farther from the box will work your glutes harder.

HAMSTRINGS AND LOWER BACK

Dumbbell Dead Lift

Another great exercise for the backs of your legs and your lower back

Standing with your feet shoulder-width apart, grasp the dumbbells and let them hang in front of your body, palms facing your thighs. With your knees straight and your head up and facing forward, slowly bend forward at the hips and lower the dumbbells along the front of your legs until you feel your hamstrings completely stretched. Contract your glutes as you raise yourself back to the starting position.

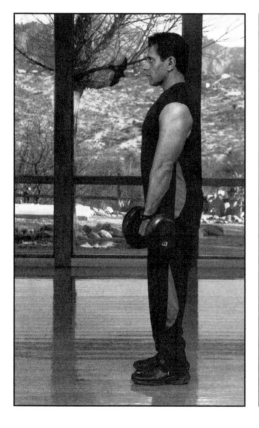 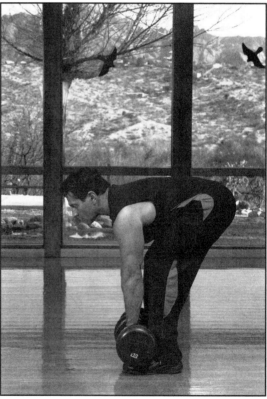

Nordine's Mindful Tip: Always keep your back straight when you are bending your knees.

THIGHS

Side-Lying Leg Abduction (Ankle Weights)

Shapes and tones the outside of your thighs

Lie on your side on an exercise mat with ankle weights on both legs. Bend your bottom leg at a 90-degree angle directly under your top leg, which should be straight. Lift your top leg up as far as possible. Complete all repetitions on one side, then switch legs and repeat on the other side.

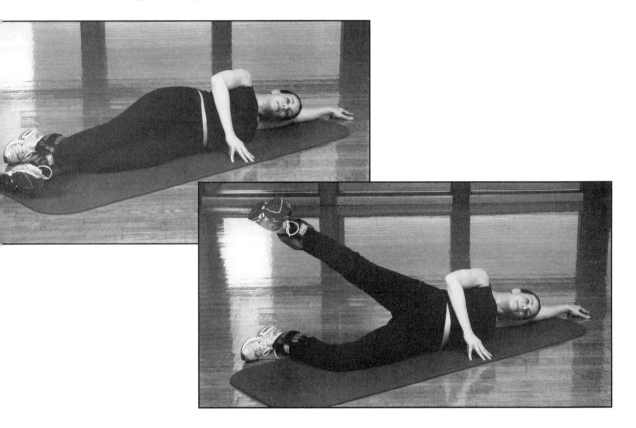

Nordine's Mindful Tip: Do not fling your leg upward; keep your movement controlled. Do not arch your back or look toward your legs while performing this movement, as this could cause stress on your neck and lower back.

THIGHS

Side-Lying Leg Adduction (Ankle Weights)

Shapes and tones inner thighs

Lie on your side on an exercise mat with ankle weights on both legs. Keep your bottom leg straight and your top leg crossed over it. Lift your bottom leg up as far as possible. Complete all repetitions on one side, then switch legs and repeat on the other side.

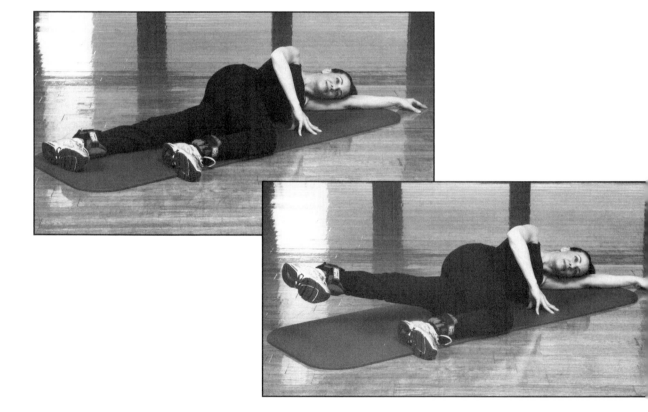

Nordine's Mindful Tip: Do not arch your back or look toward your legs while performing this movement. Doing that could cause stress on your neck and lower back.

CALVES

Dumbbell Sitting Heel Raise

Works your inner calves

Sitting on a bench with your toes on a board and your heels on the floor, hold on to a dumbbell placed across your lower thighs and rise up on your toes as high as possible.

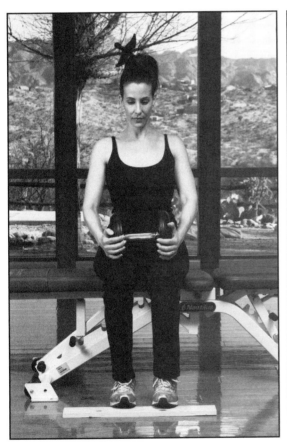 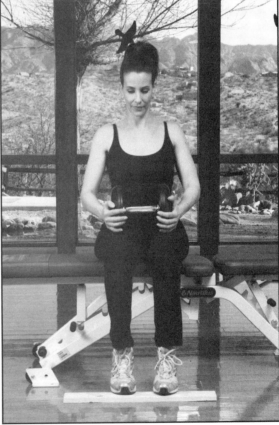

Nordine's Mindful Tip: Always keep your back straight. Avoid leaning forward with your upper body.

Stretches

Here are the three keys to proper stretching.

- Work into your stretch slowly. Don't bounce! Breathe in deeply through your nose.
- Hold your stretch for 15 seconds to give your muscles time to loosen up.
- As you complete your stretch, exhale through your nose, which will give you a deeper, more complete freedom of motion.

Upper Body Stretches

Abs Stretch

Lie facedown on a mat, toes pointed, arms bent, and palms down, just below your shoulders. Exhale as you extend your arms, raising your body and keeping your head in line with your spine. You will feel mild tension through the abdominals. Hold the position for 15 seconds.

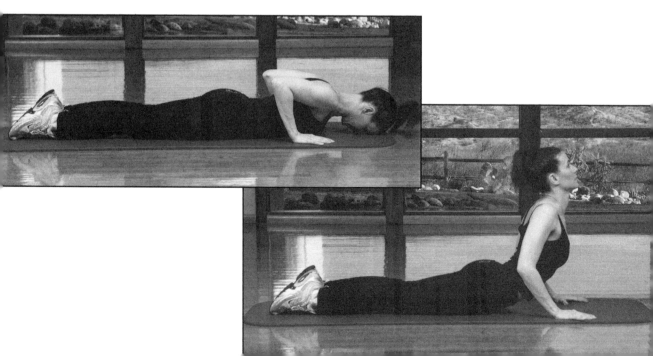

Chest Stretch

With your hands on the small of your back, arch your back until you feel the stretch. Hold the position for 15 seconds.

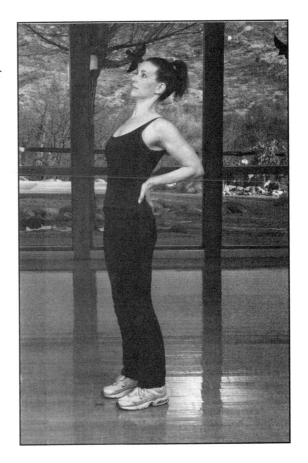

Lats (Upper Back) Stretch

Kneeling on an exercise mat, slide your hands forward and keep your buttocks back. Hold the position for 15 seconds.

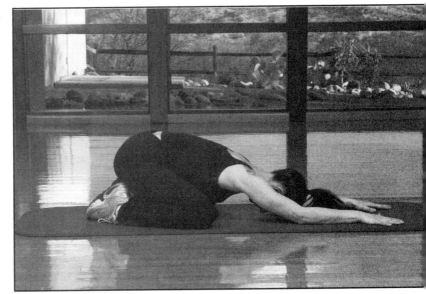

Shoulder Stretch

Pull one arm across your chest until you feel the stretch. Turn your head away from the pull. Hold the position for 15 seconds. Repeat with the other arm.

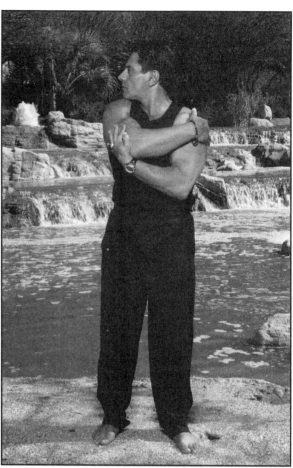

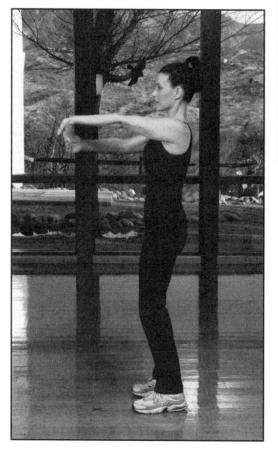

Biceps Stretch

Stretch one arm out in front of you with your elbow straight and your palm facing away. With the other hand, pull your fingers backward until you feel the stretch on the underside of your forearm. Hold the position for 15 seconds. Repeat with the other arm.

Triceps Stretch

Bend one arm behind your head and push your elbow down with the other hand until you feel the stretch. Hold the position for 15 seconds. Repeat with the other arm.

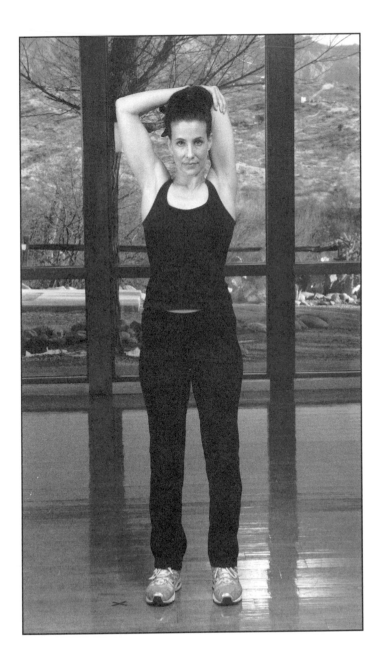

Lower Body Stretches

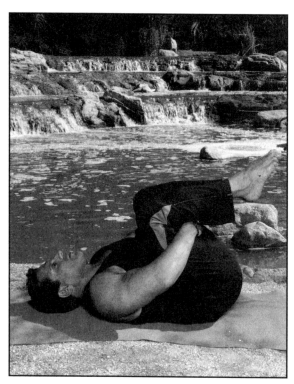

Glutes Stretch

Lie on an exercise mat with your knees bent and your feet flat on the floor. Keeping your feet and knees close together, lift your feet off the floor as you reach around your knees with your hands and hug them to your chest while keeping your back flat on the floor. Hold the position for 15 seconds.

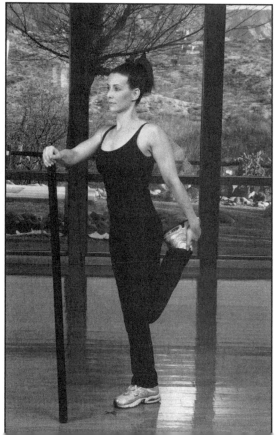

Thigh Stretch

Standing and holding on to a fitness bar or a wall with one hand for support, use your other hand to pull your heel toward your buttocks until you feel the stretch in your thigh. Hold the position for 15 seconds. Repeat with your other heel.

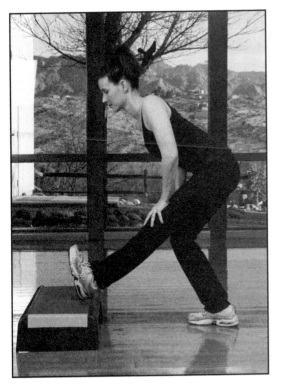

Hamstring, Lower Back, and Glutes Stretch

With one heel on a box or a step, lean forward with your hand on your knee until you feel the stretch. Hold the position for 15 seconds. Repeat with the other foot.

Calf Stretch

Holding a fitness bar or with your hands against a wall, stand with one leg in front of the other. Keeping your back leg straight, with your heel on the floor and turned slightly outward, lean forward until you feel the stretch in your calf. Hold the position for 15 seconds. Repeat with the other leg.

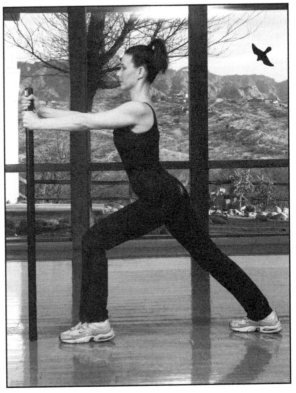

Watch Out for Symptoms of Overtraining

You need to be aware of how you feel in order to determine if you are overtraining. What's too much for you may be just right or too little for the next person. The only one who can know how you feel is you!

Here are some of the most common warning signs of overtraining.

- Loss of appetite
- Increased irritability
- Pain in the muscles or joints
- Lack of energy
- Insomnia
- Headaches
- Inability to relax
- Increased thirst, dehydration
- Lack of desire to work out (assuming you had the desire in the first place)
- Increased incidence of injury

If you are experiencing several of these symptoms at once, you should see your doctor to rule out any potentially serious cause. Otherwise, just take a few days off to rest. Drink plenty of fluids and adjust your diet if necessary. If you don't get massages on a regular basis, this would be a good time to have one or two. A good massage will help to flush toxins from your system and loosen you up if your muscles are overworked and/or tense. Get plenty of sleep and resume your workouts when you feel mentally and physically able.

Treat Yourself to a Massage

Many spa-goers, professional athletes, and fitness buffs know that a massage is relaxing, but it can be much more than that. A good massage can help increase your strength and muscle tone and speed up recovery from workouts, competitions, even injuries.

Many of us are aware that we carry tension in our neck and shoulders. Some of us have old injuries that restrict our range of motion. Still others work at jobs requiring repetitive movements, such as typing at a computer keyboard, that result in sore, fatigued muscles. When muscles tighten up because of stress or overwork, the blood flow to those muscles decreases. A massage can increase the flow of blood and nutrients to the muscles, which translates to greater strength and muscle tone.

I recommend that you treat yourself to a massage on a regular basis to reward both your body and your mind for all your good work.

Every Twelve Weeks, Give Yourself a Vacation

Every three months, take a week off from your training. Taking time off will actually allow your body and mind to come back stronger and with more determination.

In the previous chapter, I recommended that you reward yourself with a "cheat day" as you reach a new plateau every two to three weeks, not only so that you can enjoy the process but also because it will help to boost your metabolism. The principle here is the same—your vacation will be a time to rejoice in your progress and give your body time to rest.

Add Flexibility and Core Strength to Your Workout

Clients often ask me whether doing Pilates or yoga is as effective as doing strength training. My answer is that for improving muscle tone and promoting fat loss, a combination of strength training and cardiovascular exercise works best. Pilates and yoga can, however, enhance your workouts by increasing flexibility and core strength. Pilates is a technique that revolves around using a series of controlled movements designed to improve the strength and flexibility of your body. Being flexible increases your range of motion, which in turn helps your muscles function better and decreases your chances of injuring yourself. Both yoga and Pilates also engage both your mind and your body.

Take Fitness with You Wherever You Go

Many of us lead peripatetic lives, and some of my clients have bemoaned the fact that they seem to be on the road more than they're at home and don't know how to stick to a fitness routine. I understand that when you're traveling, particularly for business, you may not be able to complete the full 12/12 × 5 workout, and that's okay. Just try to do at least a few minutes of strength and cardio training every day. Here are a few tips for helping you to do that.

- **Plan ahead.** If you're going out of town, try to find out what workout facilities might be available at your hotel, whether the hotel can recommend a gym that's close by and willing to give you a daily rate, or whether there is a park or jogging track you can use.
- **Buy a set of inflatable dumbbells.** You can purchase collapsible plastic dumbbells that weigh practically nothing and take up almost no room in your suitcase. When you arrive at your destination, you simply fill them with water to achieve the desired weight, then empty them when you're ready to move on.
- **Be creative.** Instead of sticking with your normal routine, try something fun such as biking, hiking, waterskiing, rock climbing, or beach volleyball— depending on the weather and the season.
- **Try out your travel routine while you're still at home.** If you're going to be doing something different on the road, it may take more time at first, so it's a good idea to familiarize yourself with the routine before you leave home. That way, you'll avoid the frustration that could turn into an excuse not to work out at all.

Keep the Flame Burning

If you think that exercising is boring, difficult, or something you'd just rather skip, I've got news for you: sometimes I feel that way, too. That's when you can call on the techniques you've learned for using the power of your mind to change your body.

Return to your visualizations to remind yourself how you'll look and feel when you've reached your fitness goal. Affirm that you can do it, and remember the reason you're doing it—to achieve your true core desire.

When I find myself wanting to skip a workout, I use what I call the tae kwon do method of shifting my thoughts: acknowledge, accept, and let go. The basis of tae kwon do is to vanquish your opponent (in this case, your lazy or negative thought) by grabbing him (acknowledging), pulling him toward you (accepting), and throwing him to the side (letting go). When you throw your negative thought to the side, you'll make room in your mind for a positive thought to replace it. By doing that, you're adding fuel to the fire of your passion.

What fuels your passion may be different from what fuels mine. For me, it's making myself stronger and more energetic so that I know I can take care of myself and my family. To take care of others, I first have to take care of myself. If you remember what's fueling your true core desire, you'll find the source of your passion so that you can use it to keep your flame burning bright.

Seven

A Total Workout for Body, Mind, and Spirit

You can be, do, or have anything you want. If you see it in your mind, you will hold it in your hand.

I'm offering you this special thirty-minute program at the conclusion of *Mind Over Body* because it so perfectly brings together all the techniques you've been learning and embodies all the principles of living a life that is balanced in body, mind, and spirit. I developed the program a few years ago while visiting my spiritual teacher, Yogi Bhajan, in Espanola, New Mexico. It includes meditation, elements of Kundalini yoga to stretch the spine and release spiritual energy to the brain, strength training for the upper and lower body, cardio kicks, ballet stretches, and relaxation techniques.

The response I've received to this program at Miraval has been incredibly positive. One guest commented, "This is not your typical fitness class; it gets deeper into your soul and left me so connected that I won't disconnect again."

It's not intended to be a substitute for the exercise plan in the previous chapter. Rather, it's meant to supplement your regular fitness routine. I suggest that you use it when you're feeling anxious, when your energy seems to be low either mentally or physically, or when you simply want to reinvigorate the commitment you've made to yourself to live happier and healthier from now on. Do it on one of your rest days, during a workout "vacation," or simply when you want a change in your regular routine. I think you'll find that the program leaves you feeling more balanced and in touch with yourself as you go forward.

Complete the following components in the order they are presented.

Kundalini Yoga (breathing exercises for releasing spinal energy): 5 minutes

Kundalini, which was introduced to the Western Hemisphere by Yogi Bhajan in 1969, is considered the mother of all yoga styles. It focuses on awakening the energy of consciousness (Kundalini), which is found at the base of the spine. Anatomically, the spine is the link between the brain and the body. Kundalini increases oxygen and blood flow to the brain and reduces the levels of stress-related hormones such as adrenaline and cortisol. The result is that it leaves you feeling more peaceful, in control, and self-confident. The breathing exercises that follow are brought to you courtesy of Dr. Dharma Singh Khalsa.

1. Sit in a chair or comfortably cross-legged on the floor. Grab your knees (if in a chair) or your ankles (if on the floor) and take a deep breath. Flex your spine forward and lift your chest up. Exhale while flexing your spine backward. Keep your head straight so that it doesn't flip-flop. Repeat the exercise for 1 minute.

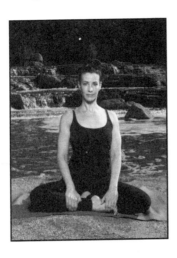 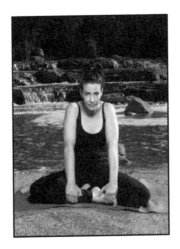

2. Grasp your shoulders so that your fingers are in front and your thumbs in back. Inhale as you twist to the left; exhale as you twist to the right. Make sure to breathe long and deep. Repeat the exercise for 1 minute. At the end, inhale and then exhale as you face forward.

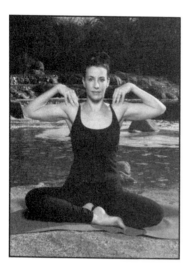 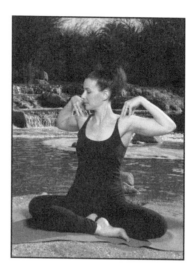

3. With your arms straight, grasp your knees firmly and, keeping your elbows straight, begin to flex your upper spine with the same movement as in exercise 1. Inhale as you flex your upper spine forward; exhale as you flex it backward. Repeat the exercise for 1 minute.

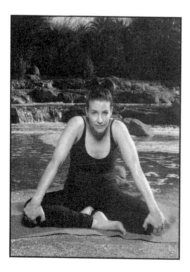 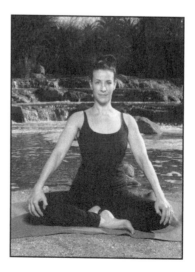

4. Pull your shoulders up toward your ears as you inhale and move them downward as you exhale. Do this 4 times. At the end, inhale and hold your shoulders pressed upward for 15 seconds, then exhale and relax them downward.

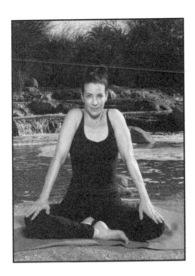 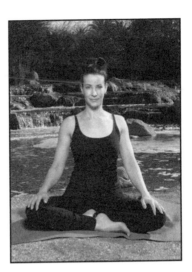

5. Roll your neck slowly to the right 3 times, then to the left 3 times. At the end, inhale facing forward. Then exhale and relax.

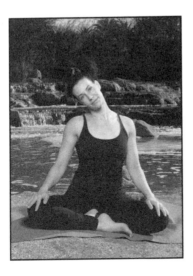 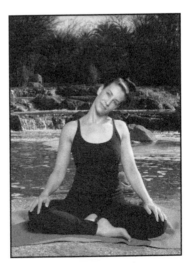

6. Stretch your arms over your head with all your fingers except your index fingers intertwined. Point both index fingers straight up. Pull your navel in as you say "sat," then relax it as you say "nam." (*Sat nam* means "my true identity.") Repeat the exercise for 1 minute. At the end, inhale as you contract your navel and direct the energy from the base of your spine up to the top of your skull.

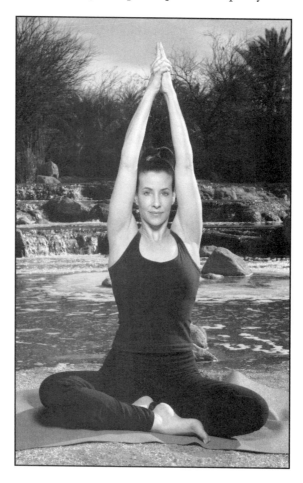

Meditation: 5 minutes

Meditation works in conjunction with Kundalini yoga to focus the mind and increase positive energy. When you do this exercise, make sure you're in a quiet, comfortable place where you won't be interrupted. Sit either on the floor or in a chair, but try to sit up straight.

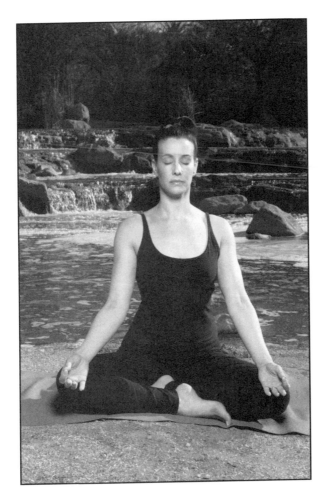

1. Close your eyes and begin to clear your mind of all conscious thoughts. When thoughts intrude, as they will, let them go.

2. Breathe slowly and deeply. Remind yourself that you are a sacred part of the universe.

3. As you continue to breathe slowly and deeply, begin to focus on your immediate environment. Listen to the sounds around you; be aware of the air touching your skin, the taste in your mouth, the smells that enter your nose.

4. Pay attention to all sensations equally. None is more important than any other. Neither embrace nor reject any of them. Detach yourself from all judgment.

5. As you begin to feel increasingly strong and centered, inhale deeply. Stretch your arms out straight in front of you and stretch your thumbs out and away from your fingers.

6. Open your eyes and focus on the tip of your nose. Breathe deeply through your nose and follow your breathing for about 1 minute. Find any tightness or tension still remaining in your body and let your peace of mind and spirit wash it away.

Once you've done 5 minutes of Kundalini yoga followed by 5 minutes of meditation, your mind will be focused, your body will be primed, and you will able to achieve the greatest benefit from the exercises that follow.

Upper Body Strength Training: 5 minutes

This part of the workout uses six of the upper body exercises in your regular strength-training routine.

- Before you begin, warm up by walking in place for 10 seconds while moving your arms in circles.
  - Do the exercises in the order they are listed.
  - Do 20 repetitions of each exercise using moderate weight. The last 3 repetitions of each exercise should be challenging, but remember that it's quality, rather than quantity, that counts.
  - Never lock your elbows.
  - Keep your navel tucked in and your feet hip-width apart when standing.
  - Have a bottle of water bottle close by and keep yourself hydrated.

Each of the following exercises is for a specific group of upper body muscles.

1. Bent-Knee Abdominal Crunch (page 140)
2. Dumbbell Incline Press (page 141)
3. Single-Arm Bent-Over Dumbbell Row (page 142)
4. Seated Dumbbell Press (page 143)
5. Standing Dumbbell Curl (page 144)
6. Bench Dip (page 145)
7. Dumbbell Triceps Kickback (page 157)

Cardio Kicks: 3 minutes

Doing 3 minutes of high-energy cardio kicks between the upper and lower body strength training segments of your routine will keep your heart at the maximum calorie-burning level while also giving you a period of "active rest."

To perform the kicks:

- Stand with your feet directly below your hips. Raise your arms over your head and bring them down as you kick upward, knee bent, first with one leg and then the other.
- Begin by doing this for just 30 seconds to 1 minute, then increase as you get used to the movement until you can do it for 3 minutes.

Lower Body Strength Training: 5 minutes

This part of the program uses six of the lower body exercises in your regular strength-training routine.

- Do the exercises in the order they are listed.
- Do 20 repetitions of each exercise using slightly more weight than you did for the upper body exercises. The last 3 repetitions of each exercise should be challenging, but remember that it's quality, rather than quantity, that counts.
- Never lock your knees.
- Keep your navel tucked in and your feet hip-width apart when standing.
- Have a bottle of water bottle close by and keep yourself hydrated.

Each of the following exercises is for a specific group of lower body muscles.

1. Dumbbell One-Leg Standing Heel Raise (page 151)
2. Reverse Crunch (page 158)
3. Dumbbell Step Up (page 159)
4. Dumbbell Dead Lift (page 160)
5. Side-Lying Leg Abduction (Ankle Weights) (page 161)
6. Side-Lying Leg Adduction (Ankle Weights) (page 162)

Ballet Stretches: 2 minutes

I call this segment ballet stretches because I want you to feel as if you are dancing with your soul while performing the movements. In my classes, I use a piece of music by Dreamcatcher called *Secret Garden* that really lifts the spirit. You feel as if your entire being is flowing with the universe.

On a practical level, the reasons for doing these stretches close to the end of your workout are as follows:

- They are a great way to cool down.
- They calm both your body and your mind and help lower your heart rate so that the relaxation segment that follows will be effective and renewing.
- They are a way to nurture your body and mind after a strenuous total workout.

Hold the position for each of the following exercises for a minimum of 10 seconds. Do not swing or bounce as you stretch.

1. Abs Stretch (page 164)
2. Chest Stretch (page 165)
3. Lats (Upper Back) Stretch (page 165)
4. Shoulder Stretch (page 166)
5. Biceps Stretch (page 166)
6. Thigh Stretch (page 168)
7. Hamstring, Lower Back, and Glutes Stretch (page 169)
8. Calf Stretch (page 169)

Relaxation: 5 minutes

For this portion of the workout, I recommend that you have three things: a yoga mat, candles (if possible), and a piece of relaxing, soothing music. I happen to like the Irish singer Enya, but you should choose whatever works for you. For more suggestions, see Further Resources (pages 187–188).

To perform the relaxation exercise, follow these steps.

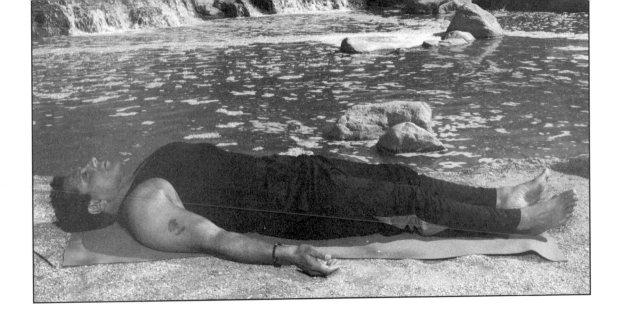

1. Lower yourself slowly onto the mat and lie with your arms at your sides and your legs slightly apart.

2. Close your eyes and take a deep breath, squeezing every muscle you're aware of as tightly as you can.

3. Exhale while relaxing your muscles.

4. With your eyes still closed, go deep within yourself, searching for your body-mind connection.

5. Pay attention to your breathing and connect—just connect. You are now one with your body, mind, and spirit.

6. After a few minutes, bring yourself back to the present by slowly opening your eyes and staring at the first thing you see. Inhale one more time—long, deep, and slow.

7. Exhale and slowly prepare to stand by rolling onto your side and using your hand to help you rise from the mat.

8. Finish in a standing position with your hands together at the level of your heart and give thanks and respect to yourself and your place in the universe.

What better way could there be for you to acknowledge all that you've done to transform yourself in body, mind, and spirit? What better way to end this book?

I wish you all the peace and tranquillity, all the fitness and health that are your birthright and that live within you right now. I wish you the total fulfillment of your true, deep core desire.

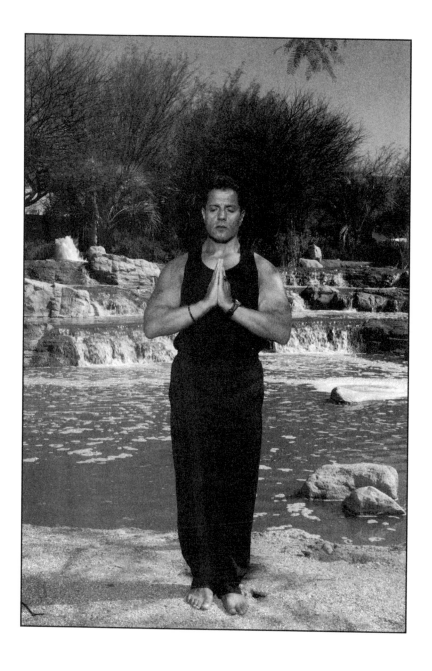

Further Resources

BOOKS TO STRENGTHEN YOUR MIND AND SPIRIT

Allen, James. *As a Man Thinketh*. DeVorss & Co., 1979.

Assaraf, John. *The Street Kid's Guide to Having It All*. Longstreet Press, 2003.

Chopra, Deepak. *The Seven Spiritual Laws of Success: A Practical Guide to the Fulfillment of Your Dreams*. New World Library, 1995.

Coelho, Paul. *The Alchemist: A Fable About Following Your Dream*. HarperSanFrancisco, 1995.

De Mello, Anthony. *The Way to Love*. Image Classics, 1995.

Hawkins, David. *Power vs. Force: The Hidden Determinants of Human Behavior*. Hay House, 2002.

Kabat-Zinn, Jon. *Coming to Our Senses: Healing Ourselves and the World Through Mindfulness*. Hyperion, 2005.

———. *Full Catastrophe Living: Using the Wisdom of Your Body and Mind to Face Stress, Pain, and Illness*. Delta, 1990.

Khalsa, Dharma Singh. *The New Golden Rules*. Hay House, 2005.

Tolle, Eckhart. *The Power of Now: A Guide to Spiritual Enlightenment.* New World Library, 1999.

Webb, Wyatt. *Five Steps to Overcoming Fears and Self-Doubt.* Hay House, 2004.

Williamson, Marianne. *A Return to Love.* Harper Paperbacks, 1996.

BOOKS FOR PHYSICAL STRENGTHENING

Anderson, Bob. *Stretching.* Shelter Publications, 2000.

DeLavier, Frederic. *Strength Training Anatomy.* Human Kinetics, 2005.

———. *Women's Strength Training Anatomy.* Human Kinetics, 2003.

Khalsa, Dharma Singh. *Food as Medicine: How to Use Diet, Vitamins, Juices, and Herbs for a Healthier, Happier, and Longer Life.* Atria, 2003.

Khalsa, Shakti Para. *Kundalini Yoga.* Perigee, 1998.

Neff, Cary. *Conscious Cuisine: A New Style of Cooking from the Kitchens of Chef Cary Neff.* Sourcebooks, 2005.

Page, Phillip, and Todd Ellenbecker. *Strength Band Training.* Human Kinetics, 2004.

Schwarzenegger, Arnold, and Bill Dobbins. *The New Encyclopedia of Modern Bodybuilding.* Simon & Schuster, 1999.

MOVIES TO INSPIRE YOU

A Beautiful Mind
Cinderella Man
The Color Purple

Dances with Wolves
Dead Poets Society
Emmanuel's Gift
Field of Dreams
Forrest Gump
Gandhi
The Green Mile
The Horse Whisperer
Iron Will
It's a Wonderful Life
Life Is Beautiful
Remember the Titans
Seabiscuit
The Shawshank Redemption
Schindler's List
Touching Wild Horses
Wild Parrots of Telegraph Hill

EMPOWERING AND RELAXING CDS AND TAPES

Anugama. *The Lightness of Being.*

Bliss. Available from www.drdharma.com.

Buddha-Bar CDs.

Chopra, Deepak. *The Soul of Healing Meditations.*

Enigma 3. *Le roi est mort, vive le roi!*

Enya. *Watermark.*

Era. *Era* and *Era, Volume 2.*

A Gift of Love: Deepak & Friends Present Music Inspired by the Love Poems of Rumi.

Kabat-Zinn, Jon. Mindfulness meditation tapes and CDs. Available from www. mindfulnesstapes.com.

Lesiem. *Illumination* and *Mystic Spirit Voices*.

Patxi. *Road to Life*. Available from www.patxi.com.

Mindful Web Sites for Body, Mind, and Spirit

www.drdharma.com. Information, insights, and products from Dr. Dharma Singh Khalsa.

www.miravalresort.com. Learn about Miraval's Life in Balance programs and more.

www.serenitysupply.com. Relaxing music therapy CDs for yoga, meditation, massage, and more.

www.tripleimpactcoaching.com, www.mindoverbodyonline.com, www.mindfulfitnessrevolution.com. Inspiration and information on Nordine's seminars, workshops, boot camps, books, DVDs, program design, online fitness coaching, fitness coaching, and fitness products.

www.yoga.com. Yoga videos and supplies.

www.zenbydesign.com. Furniture for the spirit.

Index

About the Author

Nordine Zouareg was born in the Algerian desert and taken to France by his parents as a sickly infant to receive the medical care he desperately needed to survive.

Twenty-four years later, as a champion bodybuilder, he held the titles of Mr. France, Mr. Europe, Mr. World, and Mr. Universe simultaneously. In 1995 he came to the United States as an alien of extraordinary ability and settled in Tucson, Arizona, where Dr. Dharma Singh Khalsa put him in charge of patient fitness at Khalsa International.

From Khalsa International, Nordine moved to the renowned Miraval Life in Balance spa and resort, where he managed the fitness team for five years. Since 2004 he has been Miraval's professional fitness coach, working directly with clients to identify and change the negative patterns that are preventing them from attaining optimum health and fitness.

In addition to his deep understanding of how the mind works to influence the body and his belief in the benefits of balancing body, mind, and spirit, Nordine holds a master's degree in physical education and an international personal training certification.

He lives in Oro Valley, Arizona, with his wife, Keri, and his two young children, Armand and Isabella.